Food, Nutrition and Dietetics

W0225651

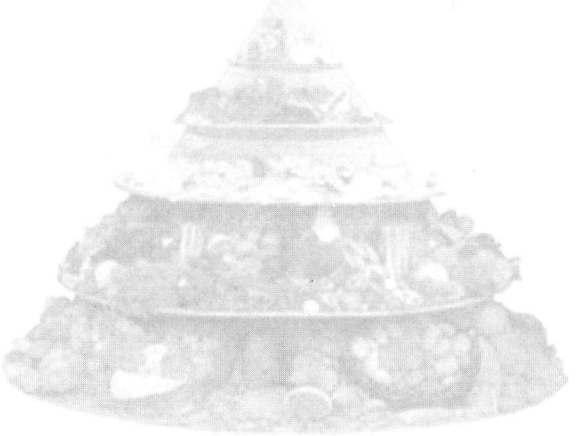

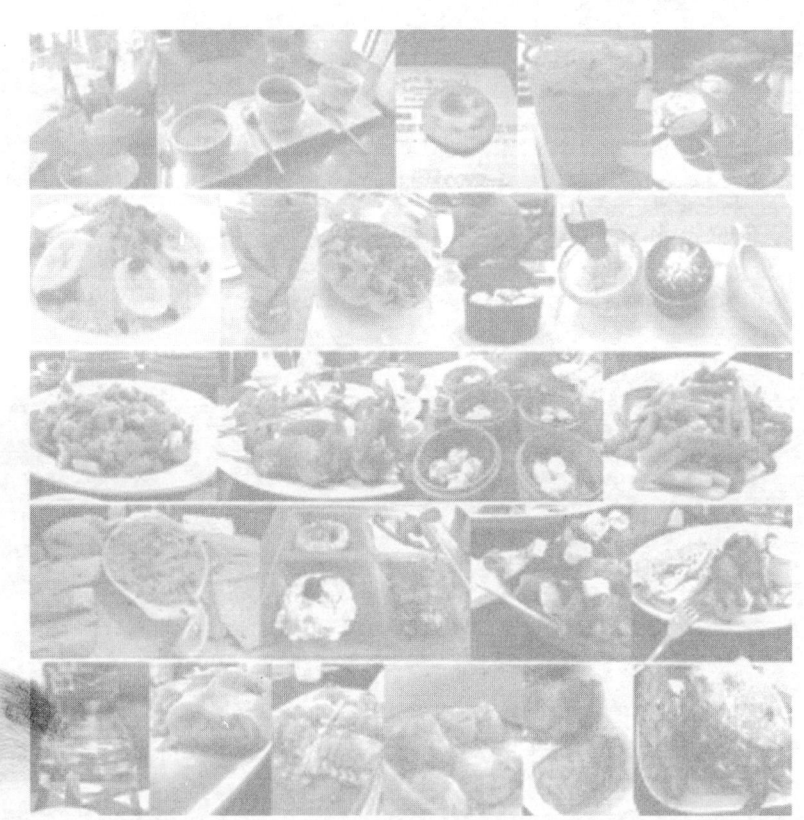

Food, Nutrition and Dietetics

Pooja Verma

MSc (Nutrition), BEd, UGC-NET/JRF, PhD Scholar

Department of Human Development and Family Studies
School for Home Sciences
Babasaheb Bhimrao Ambedkar University
(Central University)
Lucknow, UP, India

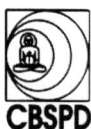

CBSPD

CBS Publishers & Distributors Pvt Ltd

New Delhi • Bengaluru • Chennai • Kochi • Kolkata • Lucknow • Mumbai
Hyderabad • Jharkhand • Nagpur • Patna • Pune • Uttarakhand

Disclaimer

Science and technology are constantly changing fields. New research and experience broaden the scope of information and knowledge. The author has tried her best in giving information available to her while preparing the material for this book. Although, all efforts have been made to ensure optimum accuracy of the material, yet it is quite possible some errors might have been left uncorrected. The publisher, the printer and the author will not be held responsible for any inadvertent errors, omissions or inaccuracies.

Food, Nutrition and Dietetics

ISBN: 978-81-239-2529-5

Copyright © Author and Publisher

First Edition: 2015
Reprint: 2018, 2023

All rights reserved. No part of this book may be reproduced or transmitted in any form or by any means, electronic or mechanical, including photocopying, recording, or any information storage and retrieval system without permission, in writing, from the author and the publisher.

Published by **Satish Kumar Jain** and produced by **Varun Jain** for

CBS Publishers & Distributors Pvt Ltd
4819/XI Prahlad Street, 24 Ansari Road, Daryaganj, New Delhi 110 002, India.
Ph: 011-23289259, 23266861, 23266867
Fax: 011-23243014

Website: www.cbspd.com
e-mail: delhi@cbspd.com;

Corporate Office: 204 FIE, Industrial Area, Patparganj, Delhi 110 092
Ph: 011-4934 4934   Fax: 011-4934 4935

e-mail: publishing@cbspd.com;
publicity@cbspd.com

Branches

- **Bengaluru:** Seema House 2975, 17th Cross, KR Road, Banasankari 2nd Stage, Bengaluru 560 070, Karnataka, India
  Ph: +91-80-26771678/79   Fax: +91-80-26771680   e-mail: bangalore@cbspd.com
- **Chennai:** 7, Subbaraya Street, Shenoy Nagar, Chennai 600 030, Tamil Nadu, India
  Ph: +91-44-26680620, 26681266   Fax: +91-44-42032115   e-mail: chennai@cbspd.com
- **Kochi:** 42/1325, 1326, Power House Road, Opp KSEB, Power House, Ernakulum Kochi 682 018, Kerala, India
  Ph: +91-484-4059061-65,67   Fax: +91-484-4059065   e-mail: kochi@cbspd.com
- **Kolkata:** 147, Hind Ceramics Compound, 1st Floor, Nilgunj Road, Belghoria, Kolkata-700056, West Bengal, India
  Ph: +033-25633055, 033-25633056   e-mail: kolkata@cbspd.com
- **Lucknow:** Basement, Khushnuma Complex, 7 Meerabai Marg (Behind Jawahar Bhawan),Lucknow-226001, UP, India
  Ph: +0522-4000032   e-mail: tiwari.lucknow@cbspd.com
- **Mumbai:** PWD Shed, Gala no 25/26, Ramchandra Bhatt Marg, Next to JJ Hospital Gate no. 2, Opp. Union Bank of India,
  Noorbaug, Mumbai-400009, Maharashtra, India
  Ph: 022-66661880/89   e-mail: mumbai@cbspd.com

Representatives

• Hyderabad	0-9885175004	• Jharkhand	0-9811541605	• Nagpur	0-9421945513
• Patna	0-9334159340	• Pune	0-9923910676	• Uttarakhand	0-9716462459

Printed at   Sanjay Printer, Sahibabad, UP, India

to
_____
my father
Shri Arvind Verma
who taught me to be
hard worker, sincere and honest

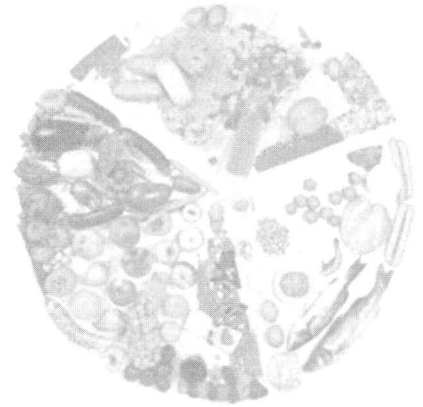

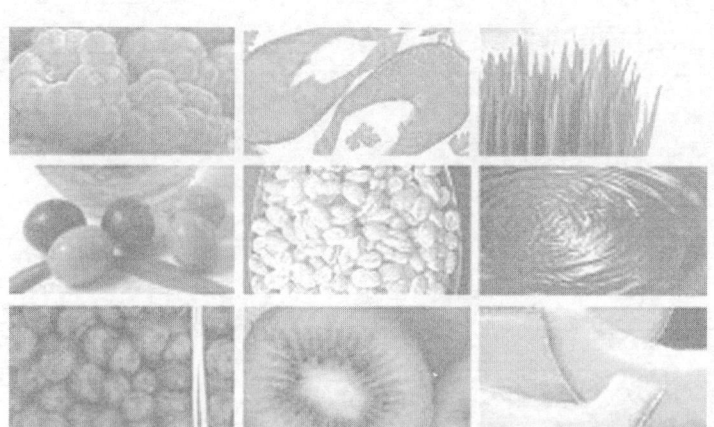

Preface

Food, Nutrition and Dietetics is the emerging field of today's era. It is a source of gaining knowledge about how to make life healthy. For humans, food is necessary for nutrition and for better nutrition, it is necessary to take the healthy diet. It is thus important to be updated regarding the knowledge of nutrition and health, and this book fulfills all these requirements.

The book covers all the key aspects of nutrition, diet and healthy preparations of the food. All the contents are written in such a way that they will help the undergraduate and postgraduate students who study home science and also the students who study nutrition at postgraduate level. The book will be helpful in finding the current text in the field of food, nutrition and dietetics. The book is updated with the latest dietary nutritional guidelines of National Institute of Nutrition (NIN), and Indian Council of Medical Research (ICMR), which are included in the Appendix. Thus, this will help the students to know about the nutritional requirements of the individuals of different age groups.

As we are living in the technical era, the lifestyle is changed and various disorders occur and our health is affected. The book deals with the healthy food preparation with modification in diet depending on the health conditions and explains the points that emphasize on preventing and minimizing the nutritional losses occurring during food preparation. The healthy tips given in between chapters will help the students in planning the diets and fundamentals of diet preparation will also be learnt.

There are also 'one word' type questions given at the end of the book which will serve as guidelines for the students who are preparing for various competitive examinations.

I am grateful to several authors, scientists, publishers of books, magazines, journals and research papers who provided very essential information and texts during compilation of the book.

My special thanks to all the teachers and professors, their blessings enabled me to write this book.

I express my sincere thanks to my parents who inspired and supported me in writing this book.

I also thank CBS Publishers & Distributors Pvt Ltd, New Delhi, for printing and giving a nice get up to the book.

Suggestions from the readers for further improvement of the content will be highly appreciated.

Pooja Verma

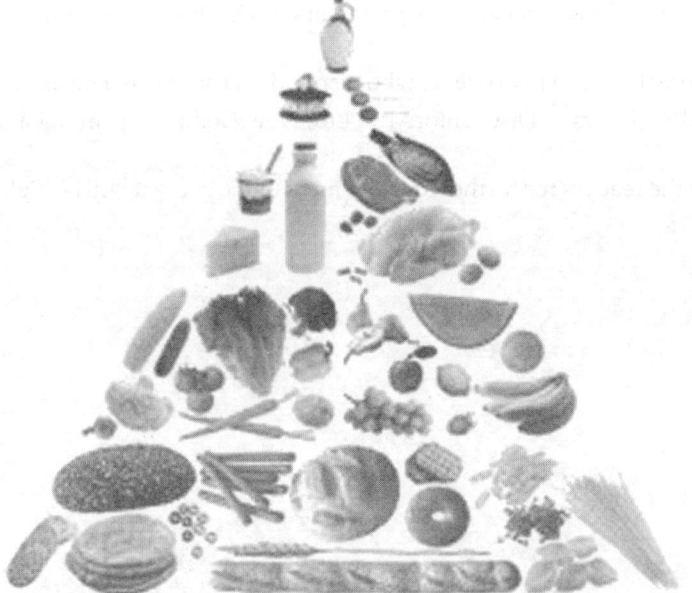

Contents

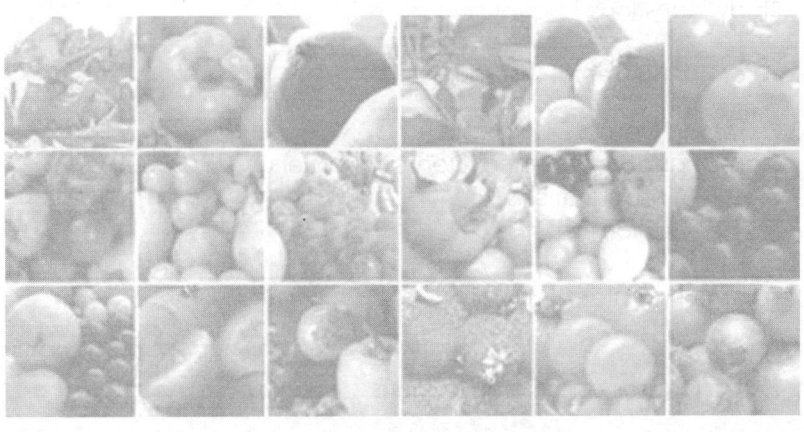

1 Nutrition and Health

Nature has gifted us very valuable things such as birds, trees, flowers, grass, animals, water and so on. Every living being for their survival depend on each other so that their life becomes possible on earth. Among all the most different and beautiful creature of God is human being. It is different in the sense of its way of living, needs and most important is its urge to change with the time.

All the living beings, whether man or animal, survive on earth due to the presence of oxygen, water and food which are very important for their existence on earth. Among all the basic requirements, food is of utmost importance and needed at all time and at every place.

Human body is complex and does various functions at every time and all the days. Each and every organ performs its activity so that we activate and work accordingly as the organs work. But how these organs work? Energy is the reason for the performance of these organs and for activation of body. Every day from morning till night we eat different food items with care and protection by thinking the beneficial aspect of the food and thinking that these will help in making us healthy and making us to feel energetic at all the time without not feeling lethargic.

Food is the most important aspect of our life. It contains various nutrients and they play very beneficial role in carrying out the important function as role of each nutrient in the body is specified and performs specific function, for example, proteins are important for growth, carbohydrates for providing energy, vitamins and minerals for carrying

out different functions. Hence food is important for health and making our life sustainable on earth.

Every individual enjoys food whether he is in a party, or at home, at the roadside or at office and schools, food is always with everyone. The food taken in balanced way and amount always makes the individual fit and strong and most important is to make them disease free. The relation of diseases and human can never be neglected. The food helps in making us fit and healthy but when any misbalancing occur in the food taken; can be harmful and disease may occur which is not good for anyone.

This is always remain a matter of concern that how the diseases or infections prevail in the body due to the food. The only reason is the mishandling or unhygienic conditions and secondly, is the improper intake of food. It is seen among the individual of middle age, the cases of cardiovascular rises or diabetes also occurs. The reason is only the improper diet or irregular dietary pattern. Therefore, it is necessary that the food should be taken accordingly with the need and at regular intervals of time. The nutritious food taken at regular interval of time lays the foundation of good health and the good health helps in spending the disease free life.

HEALTH: MEANING AND DEFINITIONS

The word **"health"** comes from the Old English word *hale*, meaning "wholeness, a being whole, sound or well." Health is regarded as the sound condition of the body which means that individual is not suffering from any kind of disease and all their duties can be performed actively by them.

Various scholars have defined health differently which are as follows:

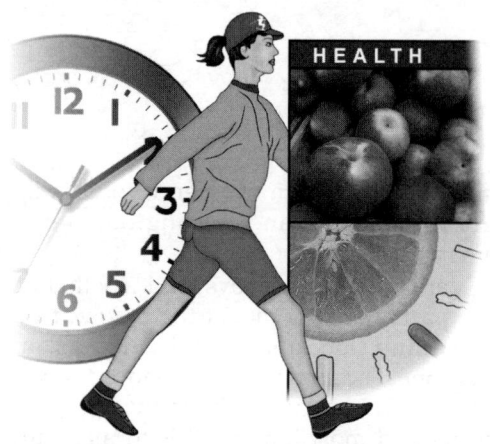

According to World Health Organization (WHO): *Health is a state of complete physical, mental and social well-being and not merely the absence of disease or infirmity.*

In Webster's 1913 dictionary, health is defined as: *The state of being hale, sound, or whole, in body, mind, or soul; especially, the state of being free from physical disease or pain.*

According to Dorland's medical dictionary, the definition of health is: *An optimal state of physical, mental and social well-being, not merely the absence of disease or infirmity.*

According to Tever: *Health is the sound stage of the individual in which his mind and body work actively.*

According to Melexicon's medical dictionary: *The state of the organism, when it functions optimally without evidence of disease or abnormality is health.*

MODERN CONCEPT OF HEALTH

With the growth of technology and advancement, the concept of health is also changed. Today the basic knowledge of health is most important. Health is believed today as the outcome of social, economic, political and environmental influences. In biomedical terms, good health is regarded as the freedom from all the diseases while in the context of other terms, health is the part of development and mere absence of disease is not the presence of good health. The health should be enjoyable, freedom from sorrows and a sound mind with sound body.

In this era, everyone has a different lifestyle and have freedom of enjoying everything in their style. Thus, health is seen as the quality of leading a good life in environment free from all sorts of discomforts and diseases.

The health is also embodiment of state of physical, mental and social well-being. These balance the integration of human with his environment, interaction with others through which the quality of life is improved, thus the individual tries to live in a happy and peaceful environment so that no bad effect on health occurs.

Types of Health

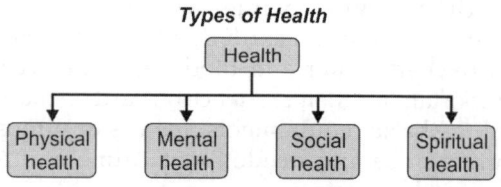

Physical health: The physical health means a body which is fit and active. The individual who works and does not feel tired readily shows that his physical health is good. The body weight, normal body size and good height are the markers of physical health.

Mental health: The cognitive and emotional well-being of an individual refers to mental health. The individual, who does not have any mental imbalance, works well and behaves well, indicates that his mental health is good. World Health Organization states that mental health is *a state of well-being in which the individual realizes his or her own abilities, can cope with the normal stresses of life, can work productively and fruitfully, and is able to make a contribution to his or her community.*

Social health: According to Donald C.A. et al. (1978), *the quantity and quality of an individual's interpersonal ties and the extent of involvement with the community* is social health.

Living with integration, sharing common thoughts with the members of society indicates the signs of good social health. One who is healthy behaves well with the other person of society and understands the necessity of others.

Spiritual health: Spiritual health includes the integrity, principles and ethics of life. The individual who is healthy do his work with sincerity and understands the concept of life.

DETERMINANTS OF HEALTH

Every individual since birth, lives in an environment, which includes everything present in the surroundings. The individual gets easily influenced by the environment. The environment of an individual helps in making the health better as well as it is also one of the reasons of making the health worse. Besides environment, there are some other factors which easily determine the health and also his society. These factors gradually interact and the health is affected.

According to World Health Organization (WHO), the main determinants of health are:

- *The social and economic environment,* i.e. our economy and society.
- *The physical environment,* i.e. where we live and what is physically around us?
- *The person's individual characteristics and behaviors,* what we are and what we do?

Our health to a great extent depends on the way of our living. The presence of good health, nutritional services, our knowledge about the health and hygiene, are also the important factors which are necessary for keeping us healthy. The other factors (determinants) that contribute towards making our health good include the following:

1. Food we eat
2. Environment in which we live
3. Physical exercise
4. Fresh air
5. Culture
6. Education
7. Genetic inheritance
8. Availability of water
9. Health services
10. Climatic conditions

Thus, the health is not only the condition of being healthy, but also in broad terms health is living disease free life or a sound condition of the body. For living a happy and prosperous life, it is not necessary to be only physically fit but one should be also fit mentally. The two aspects of health are very necessary for living a prosperous life. Man in order to enjoy and to live a successful life struggles hard which requires having power as well as capacity and the other, to have control on the emotions which will help in making the balance in life and success will be easily achieved. For making body and mind healthy, the concentration will have to be given on the diet and a well nutritionally balanced diet will help in keeping the mind and body healthy. The diet which contains all the nutrients in adequate amount helps in making physically and mentally fit and we will be able to live a disease free life.

Health is the outcome of the food consumed by us. Whatever we eat in our day-to-day life, it contributes to the health. Thus it is essential that a diet should have all the essential nutrients in right amount. For getting proper nutrients, the diet should contain different types of food in such quantities so that the need for calories, proteins, fats, minerals and vitamins are adequately met and besides these, it is also essential that enough quantities of water and fibre should also be taken so that the intestine may remain fit.

NUTRITION

The word nutrition is originated from the Latin words nutritionem and nutrire, meaning "a nourishing" or "to nourish, suckle."

Nutrition is the basic necessity of human life. He cannot be sustained without nutrition. The human being whether related to any caste, religion or any place, food is the base of everyone's life. For maintaining good health and for surviving in the environment,

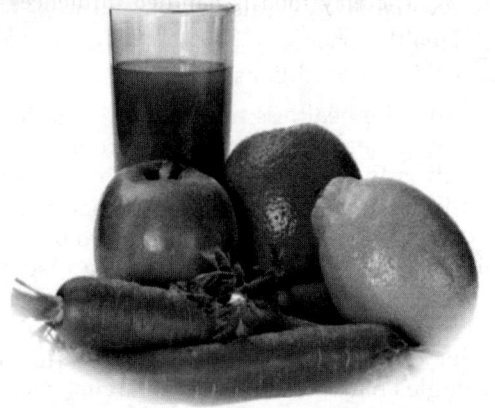

he needs food and for this he takes a nutritious diet.

It is a well known saying that *we are what we eat.* The structure and body building of an individual is easily accessed by his food, which he eats for maintaining his physical and mental healths. For being physically and mentally fit, the prime importance is given to food which ultimately leads to nutrition but the most important is to know how food helps in getting nutrition and what exactly the nutrition is?

In all the biological and chemical processes of life, *Nutrition* is involved. Nutrition starts, right from the very moment of fertilization of egg and plays an important role till the fetal development. After birth, during human growth, maturity and old age, nutrition is involved. The processes of nutrition do not stop even after death, as the human body becomes source of nutrition for other organisms. So, we can say that nutrition is an ever going process which never stops.

Everyone knows that for being healthy nutritious food is necessary. Food helps in body growth and helps in keeping the diseases away. It consists of various nutrients which help in making our body fit and strong. But, the nutrients are not easily obtained. Food has to work in the body so that each and every nutrient effects in maintenance of the body.

Thus, nutrition is the process by which living organisms take in and use food for the maintenance of life, growth, the functioning of organs and tissues; nutrition is the branch of science that studies these processes.

Nutrition is also defined as:

According to Graham Lusk; 1928: Nutrition is the scientific study of *the sum of processes concerned in the growth, maintenance and repair of the living body as a whole or of its constituent organs.*

According to Macmillan dictionary: *The science of food and its effect on health and growth* is nutrition.

According to D.F. Turner: *Nutrition is the combination of processes by which living organism receives and utilizes the material necessary for the maintenance of its functions, growth and renewal of its components.*

According to Oxford dictionary of food and nutrition: *The process by which living organisms take in and use food for the maintenance of life, growth, the functioning of organs and tissues; the branch of science that studies these processes.*

According to S. Mudambi and Shalini Rao: *The study of various nutrients, functions, food sources and their effect in human well-being is called nutrition.*

According to the American Heritage science dictionary: Nutrition is *the scientific study of food and nourishment, including food composition, dietary guidelines, and the roles that various nutrients have in maintaining health.*

In this way it is clear from the above definitions that nutrition consists of various complex processes through which body obtains energy and other vital nutrients which perform various functions for keeping body fit. When food is taken, the digestion and absorption of food occur and by the processes of digestion and absorption the nutrients are well utilized and play their specific role. The process of nutrition involves the following:

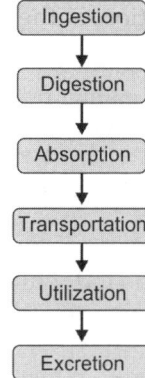

The study of nutrition deals with how these processes are involved in getting the nutrients and how the nutrients function in the body? Besides this, the study also deals with that in what amount they are needed, what are the reasons for which nutrients are needed, what are the sources of nutrients, what are the reasons of nutritional deficiencies and how they occur, what are the sources of food and what are the ways through which good nutritional status is achieved?

Basic Concepts of Nutrition

1. Nutrition is the food you eat and how the body uses it. We eat food to live, to grow, to keep healthy and well, and to get energy for work and play.
2. Food is made up of different nutrients needed for growth and health.
   - All nutrients needed by the body are available through food.
   - Many kinds and combinations of food can lead to a well-balanced diet.
   - No food, by itself, has all the nutrients needed for full growth and health.
   - Each nutrient has specific uses in the body.
   - Most nutrients do their best work in the body when teamed with other nutrients.
3. All persons, throughout life, have need for the same nutrients, but in varying amounts.
   - The amounts of nutrients needed are influenced by age, sex, size, activity and the state of health.
   - Suggestions for the kinds and amounts of food needed are made by trained scientists.

4. The way food is handled influences the amount of nutrients in food, its safety, appearance and taste.
   - Handling means everything that happens to food while it is being grown, processed, stored, and prepared for eating.

Source: Inter-agency committee on nutrition education, agricultural research service, U.S. Department of Agriculture, nutrition program news, Sept.–Oct. 1964.

The other concept of nutrition emerged in recent years is that the nutrition is very much influenced by the socio-economic development. Today the nutritional problems are also studied in terms of knowledge, living pattern, agricultural and rural aspects. It is now thought that the integrated approach must be adopted to tackle the nutritional problems and thus these concepts must be kept in mind.

Importance of Nutrition in Life

Everyone eats food according to his likings, choices and mood. Due to prolong work body gets tired and there arises a need of energy to start or to accomplish the tasks, food is required. The food we eat provides energy but it is not only needed to provide energy. The basic and important point of the thought is, why good nutrition is important?

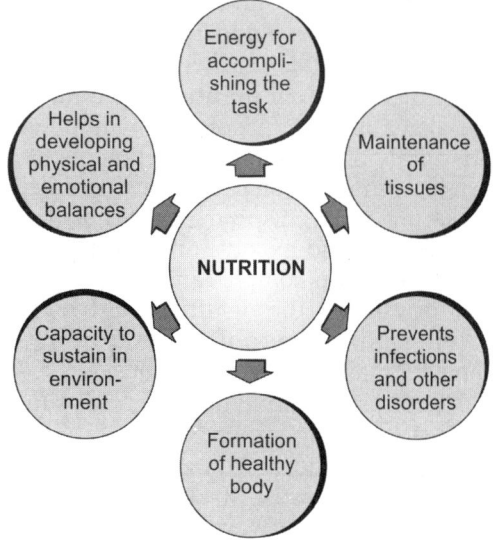

Nutrition is important because our body is formed of various cells and tissues which are needed to be maintained at regular interval of time. In the absence of good nutrition the development of body does not occur properly. The body becomes prone to get the diseases easily and nutritional disorders like night blindness, scurvy, anemia, bone disorders, etc. may also occur. Due to improper nutrition the body becomes weak which results in feeling lethargic, mottled teeth, lack of energy, lack of interest in doing the activities, low immunity, dry hairs and skin. The improper diet lacking the important nutrients results in loss of internal and external power and the body function also retards.

Although, good nutrition helps in maintaining the body functions and the essential components such as proteins, carbohydrates, fats, minerals and vitamins play important role in maintaining the structural integrity of the cells, but besides these nutrients there are some other nutrients which are also obtained from food and helps in preventing the breakdown of tissues and also prevents free radical formation. These components are phytochemicals and antioxidants which have anti-inflammatory effects and prevent damage of cells from sun, pollution, smoke and from other, such as poor food intake. Good nutrition also prevents stress and helps in digestion and absorption of food and the nutrients through the bloodstream are adequately circulated in body and are utilized whenever needed.

Besides nurturing the body, good nutrition has also a direct effect on our mental health. The ability of our mind to function well is the result of our nutritional intake. Good nutrition makes the mind fit and makes us able to take the decision and to solve out our day-to-day problems. Life is complex and full of struggles and doubts so the healthy mind helps in solving out the problems and makes us capable to take healthy decisions.

Thus, in short, good nutrition helps in:

a. Energizing out body.
b. Body building and growth
c. Maintains the structural integrity of cells
d. Develops problem solving capacity
e. Keep the diseases and infections away
f. Management of stress
g. Improves mental health
h. Develops a positive attitude towards life
i. Develops immunity

Types of Nutrition

The nutrition of an individual depends on the types of diet taken and based on this, the nutrition is of three types:

1. *Good nutrition:* When the diet taken is well balanced and rich in all amounts of nutrient as required by the individual, combining the physical activity, then the nutrition will be good.
2. *Undernutrition:* Undernutrition is the outcome of insufficient food intake that leads to the loss of weight and stunting with wasting of muscles. It can lead to reduced immunity, increased susceptibility to disease, impaired physical and mental development, and reduced productivity.
3. *Malnutrition:* Malnutrition occurs when the diet lacks the essential nutrients or when the deficiency of the nutrients occurs in the diet. The main symptoms include the loss of subcutaneous fat, dizziness, pale skin and erect hair.

RELATIONSHIP BETWEEN NUTRITION AND HEALTH

As discussed above for good health, good nutrition is very necessary. For making body healthy food taken in right amount helps in providing all the essential nutrients and performs various functions in the body.

Nutrition consists of various complex processes through which all the nutrients are utilized in the body and the health improves. The food taken at right time and in the right way creates good effect on the mind and thus the health ultimately improves. The food taken should not only be balanced but also it should be hygienic and should be served adequately.

Good nutrition helps in making body strong and develops the internal capacity so that the daily activities are carried out. The health not only depends on the way of intake but also the way of preparation is a matter of great concern. It is often seen that the food which is sold on the roadside, causes many diseases and the health is impaired. The food which is sold on the roadside or at the corner of streets is not prepared well that is the hygienic practice is not followed by the sellers, secondly the utensils which are used during the preparation of food are also becomes a source of contamination of food as they are not well washed or they are not properly kept at hygienic place and thus the microbial infection occur when the individual takes the food, the health of the individual is impaired.

Hence, the food should be kept at the hygienic places and the utensils must be thoroughly washed. As food helps in providing good nutrition and health becomes good but this is only possible when a great care will be taken in handling and serving the food in the right way. It should be always remembered that the food which will be eaten will lead to good nutrition which is necessary for good health.

FOOD GUIDE PYRAMID

A food guide pyramid is a nutrition guide which is shown in the shape of a triangle or in a shape of a pyramid. It is divided into various sections which are categorized in such a way that each section shows the recommended intake of each food group. Food Guide Pyramid was published first in Sweden, in 1974.

The main objective of the food guide pyramid is that, it helps in choosing a right diet by including the food items from each food groups. All the food items with the servings are well shown on various sections, thus it helps in making healthy choices so that diet is made balanced, by including all the food from each groups.

The United States Department of Agriculture (USDA) prepared a food pyramid, which is regarded as the important tool for choosing a healthy diet. The diet can be planned by selecting the foods which are represented graphically on the food pyramid.

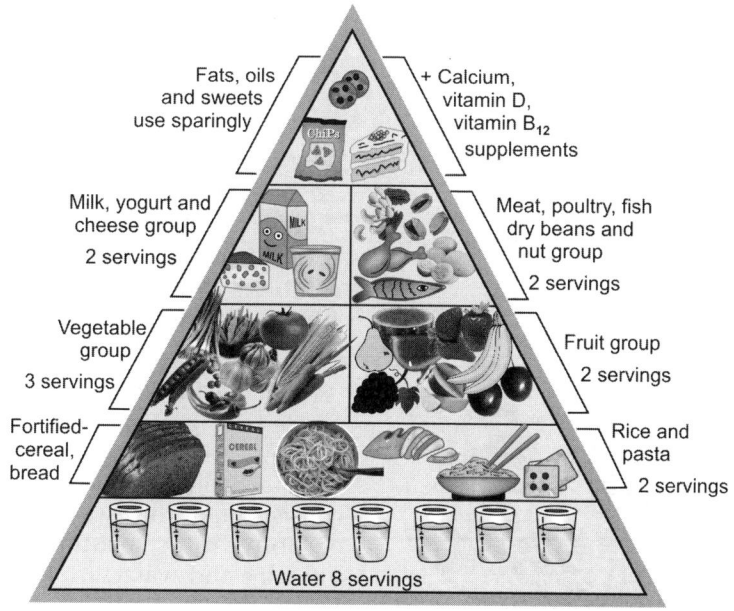

The pyramid is developed in such a way that, it helps in selecting the food items in such a way that the dietary requirements are adequately met and the level of sodium and cholesterol also remains controlled. The diet centers around the foods which are represented on the food pyramid.

The food pyramid prepared by the USDA, is shown below:

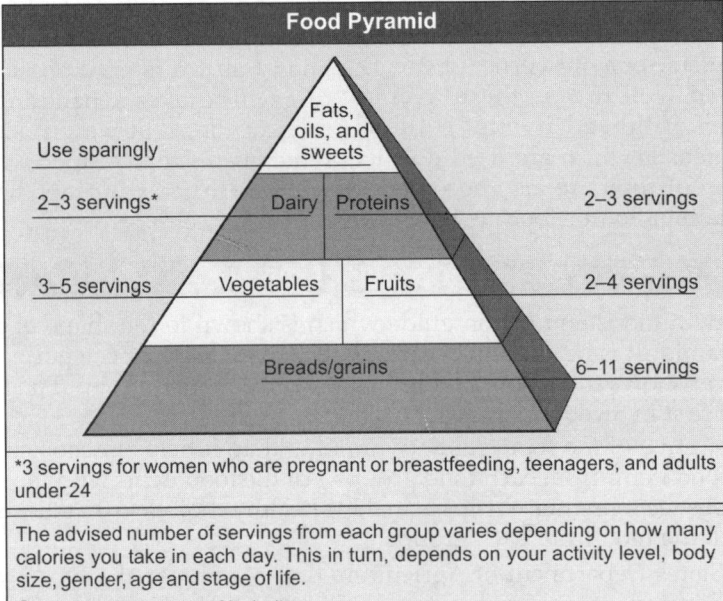

Food Pyramid

Fats, oils, and sweets — Use sparingly

2–3 servings* — Dairy | Proteins — 2–3 servings

3–5 servings — Vegetables | Fruits — 2–4 servings

Breads/grains — 6–11 servings

*3 servings for women who are pregnant or breastfeeding, teenagers, and adults under 24

The advised number of servings from each group varies depending on how many calories you take in each day. This in turn, depends on your activity level, body size, gender, age and stage of life.

Source: US Department of Agriculture

BALANCED DIET

Everyone requires food for energy and for growth and maintenance of tissues. The dietary needs of every person vary according to the age, sex and activities. Hence for getting energy and for development, a balanced diet is very necessary.

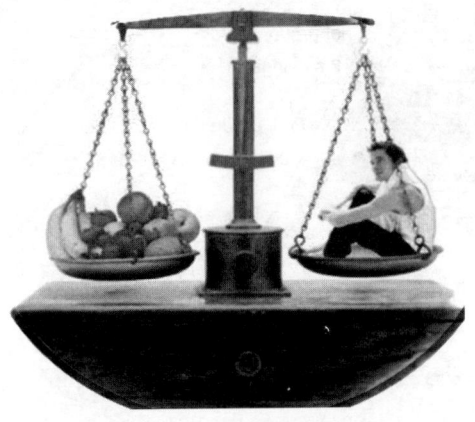

A diet that contains adequate amounts of all the necessary nutrients required for healthy growth and activity, is known as a balanced diet.

According to Dr. JS Mclester: *Balanced diet is that which both in sickness and health will meet but not exceed a person's caloric needs and which is designed to provide as far as possible in liberal excess of body's calculated requirements of all nutritive essentials, notably proteins and vitamins.*

In other words: *A balanced diet is one that contains all the nutrients needed for our body to live healthy and to do our day-to-day activities in the most efficient way.*

No single food can provide all the nutrients needed for performing the body functions well and for making everyone disease free. Only a balanced diet is a substitute, as it consists of all the essential nutrients such as carbohydrates, proteins, fats, minerals, vitamins and water, which are necessary for keeping the body fit and disease free.

Eating a balanced diet indicates that a variety of foods are selected which will help in fulfilling the nutritional needs of the individual. Balanced diet is helpful for all the age groups whether men or women. In case of women the food intake increases during pregnancy and lactation.

Need for a Balanced Diet

Balanced diet is needed because:

a. It helps in providing adequate energy needed for doing daily activities of life and for carrying out the body mechanisms correctly.

b. A balanced diet helps in maintaining the normal growth and development of body, and also repairs the damaged tissues.

c. It helps in regulation of all the body functions.

d. The nutritional requirements of the body are adequately fulfilled.

e. It helps in keeping the digestion proper and bowel movements occur well.

f. All the chemical reactions of the body occur well.

g. A balanced diet is necessary for keeping out the vitamin deficiencies which usually occur in the children of preschool period.

h. For the nourishment of all the body organs.

Table 1.1: Balanced diet as recommended by ICMR for vegetarians (the quantities are given in grams)

| Food item | Adult men | | | Adult Women | | | Children | | Boys | Girls |
	Sedentary	Moderate work	Heavy work	Sedentary	Moderate work	Heavy work	1–3 yrs	4–6 yrs	10–12 yrs	10–12 yrs
Cereals	460	520	670	410	440	575	175	270	420	380
Pulses	40	50	60	40	45	50	35	35	45	45
Leafy vegetables	40	40	40	100	100	50	40	50	50	50
Other vegetables	60	70	80	40	40	100	20	30	50	50
Root and tubers	50	60	80	50	50	60	10	20	30	30
Milk	150	200	250	100	150	200	300	250	250	250
Oil and fat	40	45	65	20	25	40	15	25	40	35
Sugar and jaggery	30	35	55	20	20	40	30	40	45	45

Table 1.2: Suggested substitution diet for non-vegetarians

Food item which can be deleted from non-vegetarian diets	Substitution that can be suggested for deleted item or items
50% of pulses (20–30 g)	1. One egg or 30 g of meat or fish 2. Additional 5 g of fat or oil
100% of pulses (40–60 g)	1. Two eggs or 50 g of meat or fish. One egg or 30 g meat 2. 10 g of fat or oil

NUTRIENTS

The food consists of a variety of chemical components which helps in growth, repairing of the tissues and regulates various body processes. Besides growth and maintenance, these chemical components help in performing various chemical reactions in the body which are essential for maintaining the health. These components are required in good amount so that the body functions well. These components are *Nutrients*.

According to Mueller and Helsel, 1996: Nutrients are chemical elements that are essential to plant and animal nutrition. Nitrogen and phosphorus are nutrients that are important to aquatic life, but in high concentrations they can be contaminants in water. These nutrients occur in a variety of forms.

Nutrients are the essential ingredients of food which nourishes the body. Food contains the various nutrients which are taken by the body in right amount. The quantity of each nutrient is fixed and the intake depends on the need of the individual. Although, they are important but overdose of the nutrients may also cause several complications.

Basically our food contains 6 types of nutrients, which are:

1. Proteins
2. Carbohydrates
3. Vitamins
4. Fats
5. Minerals
6. Water

These 6 nutrients are categorized as:

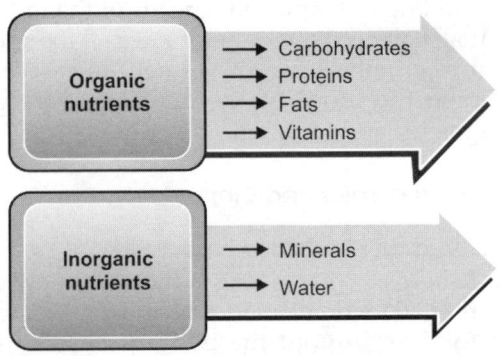

STUDY QUESTIONS

1. Define the following:
   a. Health and its types
   b. Nutrition
   c. Food guide pyramid
2. What is nutrition? Why good nutrition is important for maintaining good health?
3. What are the main factors that affect our health? Explain the relationship between health and nutrition.
4. What is the importance of nutrition in our life? What are the essential nutrients required for achieving good health?
5. Discuss the importance of balanced diet in our life.
6. What is malnutrition? What are the factors responsible for malnutrition?
7. What is food guide pyramid? How food guide pyramid is regarded as the important tool in planning meals?

2 Food

Food is the basic necessity of our life. It provides the necessary components that are needed for growth, energy and for regulation of the body activities. Food is very important for survival of human being.

With the growth and advancement the concept of food is changed. With the technical advancement it is considered that food is not the only medium of fulfilling the desire of hunger but it is also important for living a healthy and disease free life.

Food acts as the fuel of our body. We daily eat various things such as rice, apple, banana, pulses, grams, breads, sweets, meats, *etc*. The intake of the items depends on the choice and interest of individual. Thus food is defined as anything *eaten by us that provides energy, builds our body, keeps us mentally and physically fit, is food.*

Food may also be defined as *any substance consumed which provides nutritional support to the body is known as food.*

According to Usha Tandon: *Food is that which nourishes the body. Different foods are alike in their ability to nourish, because each food does not contain identical amount of nutrients.*

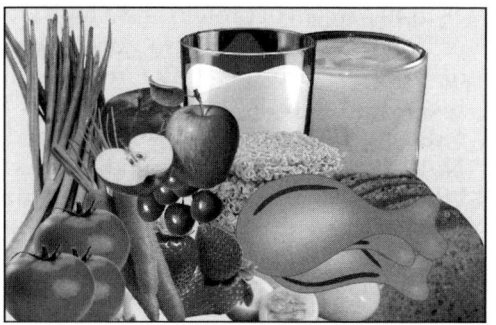

FUNCTIONS OF FOOD

Food performs various important functions in the body. The main functions of food are:

Foods provide energy: The most vital function of food is to provide energy. The food taken by us acts as fuel which provides energy and this energy is used for performing daily activities of life such as walking, running, sleeping, *etc*. The main sources of energy are carbohydrates and fats. It is necessary that all the food items containing the energy providing components should be supplied in sufficient quantity, if taken in excess then it will be stored as body fat, which will result in obesity.

Growth and maintenance: Proteins are the essential component of food which helps in maintenance of tissues. With age growth occurs which is only maintained by proteins. Besides these growth proteins are also necessary for repairing the injured tissues and cells.

Protection from infections: Minerals and vitamins are the most important constituents of food. The food taken in balanced amount provides minerals and vitamins which help in keeping the immunity strong so that infections do not occur and also these help in keeping the organ healthy.

Social functions of food: Food has always been considered as important part of our community, social, cultural and religious lives. During functions such as social parties, birthday parties, marriage ceremonies, it has been an expression of love, friendship and happiness at family and friends get-together.

Psychological functions of food: The psychological needs of the people are also satisfied by food. During special preparation of any food at any special occasion the people meet each other and shares the food, thus a sense of security and love develop among the people.

FOOD GROUPS

Daily, we eat a number of food items and the planning of our food depends on the selection of the food items. The meal is balanced in such a way that it must include each and every item so that the nutritional requirement is filled.

The daily requirement of food depends on our physical activity and other tasks performed. But the point is to remember that what types of foods are selected so that the body's requirements are well met and an adequate or nutritionally balanced diet is made. In a family the people of all age groups live, thus a diet is needed to be planned in such a way that the requirements of all members are fulfilled.

Depending on this the experts have advised such a plan, which is known as food group that means good nutrition through proper food selection.

A food group is defined as a collection of foods that are categorized according to the nutrients they provide.

The food group is a classification of all food items which are included in the diet. Food groups act as guide which helps in selecting the food when meal preparation is done.

Basic 11 food groups and their nutritive values

Based on the nutritive values foods are basically classified into 11 groups and these are:

1. **Cereals and millets:** Cereals and millets are the staple foods for a majority of our population. Cereals are good sources of proteins and vitamins. They are considered as the important source of carbohydrates, thus provides energy. The foods in this group include rice, wheat, jowar, bajra, and other products made from these such as rice flakes, vermicelli, *etc.*

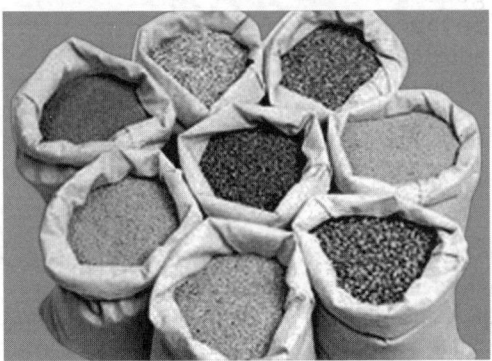

2. **Pulses:** The second group comprises all legumes which are major sources of proteins in our diet. These are contained about 20–24 percent of proteins. Besides proteins, these are also good sources of vitamins and minerals. Pulses are used in different forms and their nutritive value of pulses increases during fermentation and germination. Red gram, green gram, bengal gram and black gram are the major pulses widely used in India.

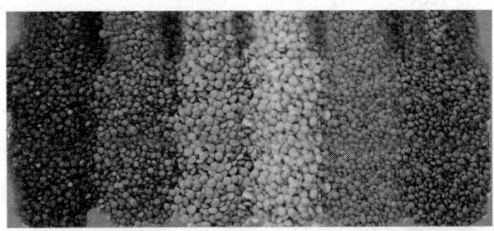

3. **Nuts and oilseeds:** Nuts and oilseeds are rich sources of proteins especially amino acid arginine. These are contained about 18 to 40 percent of protein and a high level of fat, hence these are also good sources of energy. Studies have found that inclusion of nuts in the diet helps in reducing the cholesterol level in the body. Nuts such as almonds are good sources of vitamin E and are good for preventing heart ailments.

Soyabean, is widely consumed as oil, soya sauce, soya proteins, soya nuts, soyabean flour. It is a good source of protein and contains 40% of proteins and 20% of fat. Besides proteins, soyabeans are also a good source of iron and B-vitamins. Soyabean also contains anticancerous substances such as isoflavones thus found to be protective against cancer.

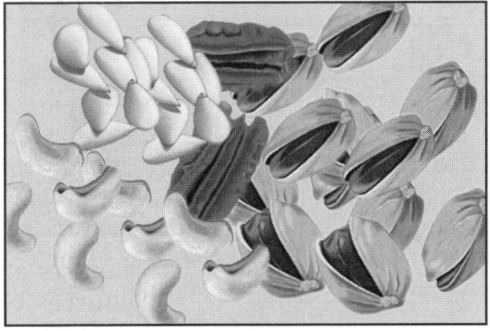

4. **Vegetables:** Vegetables are plant foods which are consumed as raw or in cooked form. Vegetables provide a variety to diet and are good sources of vitamins and minerals. Based on nutritive values, vegetables are broadly divided into three groups:
   i. Green leafy vegetables
   ii. Roots and tubers
   iii. Other vegetables

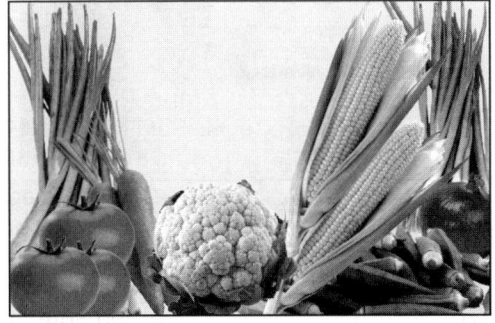

Green leafy vegetables: Green leafy vegetables are good sources of vitamins and minerals and carotenes are also present in excellent amount. Iron is another important nutrient present in greens. Green leafy vegetables need to be preserved immediately due to presence of moisture.

Roots and tubers: This group includes potato, sweet potato, tapioca, carrot, beet root, raddish and colocasia. These are good sources of carbohydrates. Carrots are good sources of carotene. Roots and tubers are poor sources of proteins and are fairly good sources of vitamin C.

Other vegetables: Brinjals, pumpkin, cauliflower, tomatoes, garlic, ginger and capsicum comes in this group. These are contained a very low amount of nutrients and contribute fibre to diet.

5. **Fruits:** Fruits are juicy and pulpy and are produced from flowers of plants. These are sweet and have aromatic flavors. Fruits are poor sources of fat and proteins. Fruits like banana are very good sources of energy. Yellow fruits are very good sources of carotenes and amla, oranges, guava are very good sources of vitamin C. Fruits contain antioxidants thus prevent many diseases.

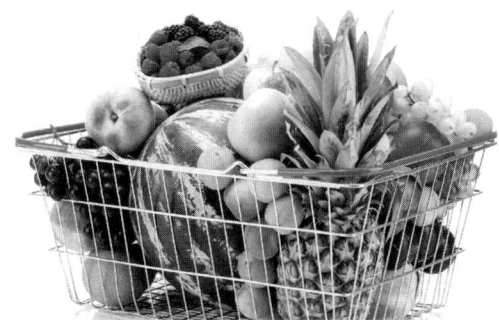

6. **Milk:** Milk is an important animal food and is considered as a complete food because of presence of all the essential nutrients which are important for growth and development. Milk contains lipids, carbohydrates, proteins and minerals and vitamins are also present in good amount. The proteins present in milk are of high biological value and the fat present in milk is easily digestible.

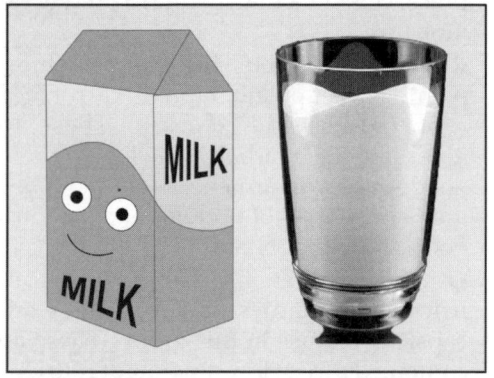

7. **Eggs:** Eggs are another animal food and are important source of proteins and other vital nutrients. The most commonly used eggs are the chicken's eggs. The eggs are the important sources of essential amino acids. It also provides vitamins like retinol (vitamin A), riboflavin (vitamin B_2), folic acid (vitamin B_9), vitamin B_6 and vitamin B_{12}. Besides vitamins, minerals such as choline, iron, calcium, phosphorus and potassium are also important components of eggs. Egg is a poor source of vitamin C.

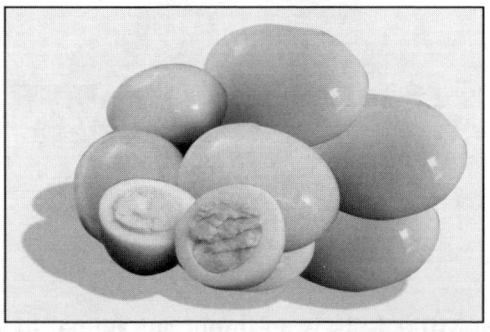

8. **Meat and meat products:** Due to presence of the proteins, meat is a very important part of diet. It is obtained by slaughtering the animals and mostly flesh of animal is consumed. The meat of cattle, sheep and pigs is mostly consumed. Meat contains proteins such as actin, myosin, collagen and elastin. The amino acids found in meat are good for growth and development. Cholesterol in meat is present in very high amount and carbohydrates are present in very lesser amount.

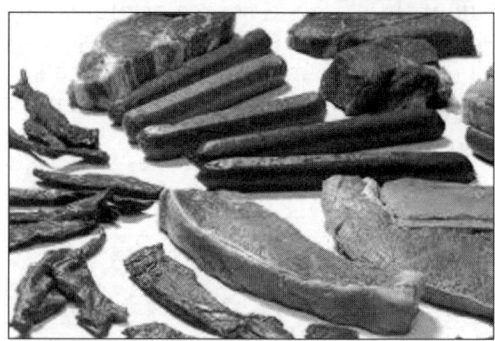

9. **Fats:** Fats and oils are the major sources of energy and are present naturally in many foods. Most oils and fats give 900 kcals per 100 grams. Fats are the excellent sources of fat soluble vitamins such as vitamin A, vitamin D, vitamin E and vitamin K and also provide the essential fatty acids.

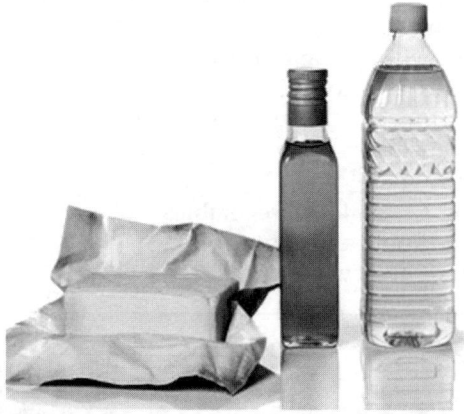

10. **Sugar and its products:** Sugar is found in most of the plant foods but its main

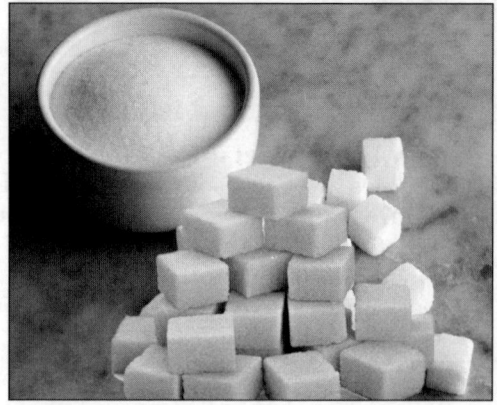

sources are sugarcane and sugar beet. It is a very good source of energy. The main products are jaggery, caramel sugar, molasses, honey, maltodextrins and corn syrup.

11. **Spices and condiments:** Spices are the plant or vegetable products that are used

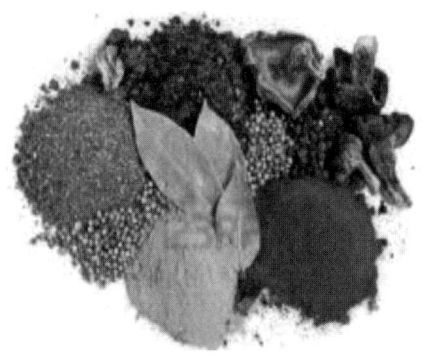

for enhancing the taste and flavor of food. Spices stimulate salivation and thus make food acceptable. Spices are good sources of antioxidants and aids in digestion. Species and condiments also have medicinal importance and helps in preventing the diseases. Common spices such as clove, cinnamon, ginger, turmeric are good sources of antioxidants and are anti-carcinogenics.

ICMR FIVE FOOD GROUP SYSTEM: Indian Council of Medical Research (ICMR) has suggested that foods are grouped into five parts and the meal preparation should include the food items from each group.

According to ICMR the five food group system is as follows:

Food group	Main nutrients
I. **Cereals, grains and products:** Rice, wheat, ragi, bajra, maize, jowar, barley, rice flakes, wheat flour.	Energy, protein, invisible fat, vitamin B_1, vitamin B_2, folic acid, iron, fibre.
II. **Pulses and legumes:** Bengal gram, black gram, green gram, red gram, lentil (whole as well as dhals) cowpea, peas, rajmah, soyabeans, beans	Energy, protein, invisible fat, vitamin B_1, vitamin B_2, folic acid, calcium, iron, fibre.
III. **Milk and meat products:** **Milk:** Milk, curd, skimmed milk, cheese **Meat products:** Chicken, liver, fish, egg, meat.	 Protein, fat, vitamin B_{12}, calcium. Protein, fat, vitamin B_{12}, calcium.
IV. **Fruits and vegetables:** **Fruits:** Mango, guava, tomato ripe, papaya, and orange, sweet lime, watermelon. **Vegetables (green leafy):** Amaranth, spinach, drumstick leaves, coriander leaves, mustard leaves, fenugreek leaves **Other vegetables:** Carrots, brinjal, ladies fingers, capsicum, beans, onion, drumstick, cauliflower.	 Carotenoids, vitamin C, fibre Invisible fats, carotenoids, vitamin B_2, folic acid, calcium, iron, fibre Carotenoids, folic acid, calcium, fibre
V. **Fats and Sugars:** **Fats:** Butter, ghee, hydrogenated oils, cooking oils like groundnut, mustard, coconut. **Sugars:** Sugar, jaggery	 Energy, fat, essential fatty acids Energy

EXCHANGE LIST SYSTEM

The exchange list is defined as a list containing the food groups in a specified amount having the essential nutrients such as carbohydrates, proteins, fats, vitamins and mineral values.

The exchange list system was developed by the American Diabetes Association in collaboration with American Dietetic Association, in 1950, to help the diabetic patients in planning their meal. Based on the similar pattern, the other countries also prepared the food list to select the food according to the need.

In India, the exchange list was prepared by major agencies working in the field of nutrition. The agency, namely the home science colleges, the dietetics department of nutrition and Indian Council of Medical Research works in the field of nutrition. The food having different nutrients and amounts, are divided into group and the food from the particular groups is chosen which is called an exchange. The exchange chosen represents the quantity or the amount having different micronutrients (Appendix-A).

STUDY QUESTIONS

1. Why food is considered as the basic necessity of life? Give definitions of food. What are the main functions of food?
2. What is ICMR's five food group system?
3. What is the importance of exchange list system?

3 Recommended Dietary Allowances

We eat daily a number of food items which enable our body to do various activities efficiently. The food we take daily provide us various nutrients which help in carrying out body functions efficiently and also makes us fit and strong. As mentioned that the food we take provide a variety of nutrients but it is also necessary to explain the amount of nutrients that is needed to be taken daily. For this the concept of recommended dietary allowances (RDAs) is originated.

The main principle behind setting up the RDA is that the people of different age and different sex have different nutritional requirements. For assuring the adequate nutritional intake the standards are set up. The standards are based on the need and requirements of the individual.

According to Indian Council of Medical Research (ICMR), recommended dietary allowance (RDA) is defined as *the average daily dietary nutrient intake level sufficient to meet the nutrient requirement of nearly all (97 to 98 percent) healthy individuals in a particular life stage and gender group.*

Thus, recommended dietary allowances (RDAs) are the levels of intake of adequate and essential nutrients necessary to meet the known nutritional needs of all healthy persons. The RDAs are used as a guide to determine the nutritional adequacy of individual diets. The RDA also covers the problems of the individual and during abnormality or during metabolic disorders the RDAs are considered so that the diet is well planned with respect to conditions of the patients. (The revised recommended dietary allowances for Indians — 2010, by NIN, (ICMR) is given in Appendix-B.)

PRINCIPLES OF DERIVING RDA

A number of methods have been employed over the years to derive the requirement of different nutrients of individuals. The general principles underlying these methods are:

Dietary intakes: Dietary intake is an important approach, which is used to determine the energy requirement of children. The energy intakes of growing children are considered to be determined for determining the nutrient level.

Growth: This approach is used during the early infancy (0–1 yr). The intake of breast milk and its nutrient composition are utilized for defining the nutrient requirement as the only mode of meeting the nutritional requirement is breast milk so growth is estimated.

Nutrient balance: The minimum intake of a nutrient for equilibrium (intake=output) in adults and nutrient retention consistent with satisfactory growth in infants and children, for satisfactory maternal and fetal growth during pregnancy, satisfactory output of breast milk during lactation have been used widely in arriving at the protein requirements.

Obligatory loss of nutrients: This approach has been widely used in assessing the protein requirement. The minimal loss of any nutrient or its metabolic product (e.g. nitrogenous end products of proteins) through normal routes of elimination, *viz.* urine, faeces and sweat is determined on a diet devoid of, or very low in the nutrient under study (*viz.* protein-free diet). These values are used to determine the amount of nutrient to be consumed daily through the diet to replace the obligatory loss of the nutrient and it represents the maintenance needs of an individual (*viz.* adults). In infants and children, growth requirements are added to this maintenance requirement.

Factorial approach: In this approach, the nutrients required for carrying out various activities such as sleep, rest, exercise, *etc.* are assessed separately and added up to arrive at the total daily requirement. The factorial approach is also the basis of computing the energy requirement.

Depletion and repletion studies: Depletion and repletion are another important approaches which are used in determining requirement of water-soluble vitamins. The level of the vitamin is determined by employing this approach. The subjects are first fed a diet with very low levels of the vitamin till the biochemical parameter reaches a low level, then response to feeding graded doses of the vitamin with the diet are determined. The level at which the response increases rapidly corresponds to the level of the requirement of the vitamin.

Nutrient turnover: The studies of turnover of nutrients in healthy persons, using isotopically labeled nutrients are employed in arriving at the requirement of certain nutrients. Requirements of vitamin A, vitamin C, iron and vitamin B_{12} have been determined employing this approach. In this approach stable isotopes, which are safer, are being increasingly used to determine the turnover of nutrients in the body.

REFERENCE BODY WEIGHT

Gender, age and weight are very important parameters of determining the nutritional requirements. These are the best indicators of the health and growth rates. The weight and height of the adult or the child are considered in recommending the RDAs so that a good physical development is attained. Besides this, the deficiency in the nutrients can also be estimated and then the anthropometric standard is well achieved.

Table 3.1: Standard heights and weights of Indians

Males			Age (years)	Females		
Weight (kg)	Height (cm)	BMI		Weight (kg)	Height (cm)	BMI
11.2	82.4	16.5	1+	10.7	81.6	16.1
13.0	90.7	15.8	2+	12.6	89.8	15.6
14.8	99.1	15.1	3+	14.4	98.2	14.9
16.5	105.7	14.8	4+	16.0	105.1	14.5
18.2	111.5	14.6	5+	17.7	111.0	14.4
20.4	118.5	14.5	6+	20.0	117.5	14.5
22.7	124.3	14.7	7+	22.3	123.6	14.6
25.2	130.1	14.9	8+	25.0	129.2	15.0
28.0	134.6	15.5	9+	27.6	135.0	15.1
30.8	140.0	15.7	10+	31.2	140.0	15.9
34.1	144.8	16.3	11+	34.8	145.3	16.5
38.0	151.1	16.6	12+	39.0	150.2	17.3
43.3	157.0	17.6	13+	43.4	153.8	18.3
48.0	163.0	18.1	14+	47.1	157.0	19.1
51.5	166.3	18.6	15+	49.4	158.8	19.6
54.3	168.3	19.2	16+	51.3	159.7	20.1
56.5	170.0	19.6	17+	52.8	160.2	20.6
58.4	171.3	19.9	18–19	53.8	161.1	20.7
60.5	172.5	20.3	20–24	54.8	160.7	21.2
62.0	172.3	20.9	25–29	56.1	161.0	21.6

Source: National nutrition monitoring bureau: Diet and nutritional status of rural population. Technical report No. 21, NIN, ICMR, 2002.

Standard heights and weights of infants and preschool children

Boys		Age in months	Girls	
Weight (kg)	Height (cm)		Weight (kg)	Height (cm)
3.3	49.9	0	3.2	49.1
4.5	54.7	1	4.2	53.7
5.6	58.4	2	5.1	57.1
6.4	61.4	3	5.8	59.8
7.0	63.9	4	6.4	62.1
7.5	65.9	5	6.9	64.0
7.9	67.6	6	7.3	65.7
8.3	69.2	7	7.6	67.3
8.6	70.6	8	7.9	68.7
8.9	72.0	9	8.2	70.1
9.2	73.3	10	8.5	71.5
9.4	74.5	11	8.7	72.8
9.6	75.7	12	8.9	74.0
10.9	82.3	18	10.2	80.7
12.2	87.8	24	11.5	86.4
13.3	91.9	30	12.7	90.7
14.3	96.1	36	13.9	95.1
15.3	99.9	42	15.0	99.0
16.3	103.3	48	16.1	102.7
17.3	106.7	54	17.2	106.2
18.3	110.0	60	18.2	109.4

Source: WHO Multicenter growth reference study group. WHO child growth standards. Height for age, weight for age, weight for height and body mass index for age. Methods and development. WHO, Geneva, 2006.

REFERENCE WOMAN AND REFERENCE MAN

Nutritional requirements vary with the age, activities and size of the body and thus for computing the total nutritional intake, the concept of reference man and reference woman is used.

Reference woman: The reference woman is defined as:

Age	18–29 yrs
Weight	55 kg
Height	1.61 m
Body mass index (BMI)	20.3

The **reference woman** is free from disease and physically fit for active work; on each working day, she is engaged in 8 hours of occupation which usually involves moderate activity, while when not at work she spends 8 hours in bed, 4–6 hours in sitting and moving about, 2 hours in walking and in active recreation or household duties.

Reference man:

Age	18–29 yrs
Weight	60 kg
Height	1.73 m
Body mass index (BMI)	20.3

The **reference man** is free from disease and physically fit for active work; on each working day, he is engaged in 8 hours of occupation which usually involves moderate activity, while when not at work he spends 8 hours in bed, 4–6 hours in sitting and moving about, 2 hours in walking and in active recreation or household duties.

Table 3.2: Reference body weights of Indians of different age groups

Groups	Age	Reference body weight
Adult man	18–29 yrs	60.0
Adult woman	18–29 yrs	55.0
Infants	0–6 months	5.4
	6–12 months	8.4
Children	1–3 yrs	12.9
	4–6 yrs	18.0
	7–9 yrs	25.1
Boys	10–12 yrs	34.3
	13–15 yrs	47.6
Girls	10–12 yrs	35.0
	13–15 yrs	46.6

Source: WHO multicenter growth reference study group. WHO child growth standards. Height for age, weight for age, weight for height and body mass index for age. Methods and development. WHO, Geneva, 2006.

Table 3.3: Classification of activities based on occupation

	Male	Female
Sedentary	Teacher, tailor, barber, executive, shoemaker, housewife, priest, retired, personnel, landlord, peon, postman, computer professional	Teacher, tailor, computer professional, executive, housewife.
Moderate	Fisherman, basket maker, potter, goldsmith, maid, coolie, basketmaker, agricultural labour, carpenter, mason, rickshaw puller, beedi maker, electrician, fitter, turner, welder, industrial labour, coolie, weaver, driver, servant	Maid, coolie, basket maker, agricultural labour, beedi maker.
Heavy	Stone cutter, blacksmith, mineworker, wood stone cutter	Stone cutter

Source: Modified. Gopalan, C, Ramasastri BV and Balasubramanian SC (1991). Nutritive value of Indian foods, National institute of nutrition, ICMR, Hyderabad, India.

USES OF RDA

The RDA of nutrients is used for a number of purposes. They are:

1. To predict food needs of the individual.
2. To help the government in framing the nutritional policies according to the need of the persons.
3. To help in modifying the diet according to the physical and mental conditions of the individual.
4. To help in achieving the good nutritional status.
5. To guide the planner in planning the nutritionally adequate meal.
6. To help in understanding the nutritional requirements so that well planning of diet is done.
7. To evaluate the results of surveys.
8. To formulate the policies on the basis of nutritional needs at the national level.
9. To establish guidelines for labeling of food from the nutritional standpoint.
10. To develop nutrition education programmes.

FACTORS AFFECTING RDA

1. *Age*: RDAs vary according to the age of the individual. For instance an infant requires more protein per kilogram of body weight than adolescent, since their metabolic rate is much faster than that of adolescent.
2. *Sex*: The needs of male and female also vary. Due to the physiological differences the RDAs differ. Adolescent girls require more iron than adolescent boys in order to replace iron lost during menstruation on every month.
3. *Body size*: The individuals who are tall and are heavy need more calories than the individuals who are small statured man, since their body surface area is more.
4. *Physical state*: The quantity of proteins and other nutrients increases during

pregnancy and pregnant women requires more nutritious food than ordinary adult women, since they have to meet the additional nutritional requirements of the growing foetus. Similarly the woman who breastfed her baby have increase nutritional requirements.

5. *Types of work*: A sedentary worker requires less calories than a heavy worker, since the sedentary expends less energy than moderate and heavy, during work.

STUDY QUESTIONS

1. What do you mean by RDAs?
2. What are the main principles of deriving RDAs for different age groups?
3. What are the main parameters of determining nutritional requirements?
4. Give answers of the following:
   - Reference men and women
   - Uses of RDAs
   - Classify the activities based on occupation of an individual.

4 Meal Planning

Meal planning is the most important aspect which involves the careful investigation of the food items present and what is needed to be purchased?

In the context of health and nutrition, meal planning requires the inclusion of all the food items which are needed to meet the nutritional requirement of the individual. Meal planning is important because it ensures that a careful planned meal will help in meeting all the requirements of the health and secondly it will help in saving the energy and money.

The most important criterion of the meal planning is the number of members present in the family. As there are different family members having different ages thus the nutritional requirements also vary. Thus, it is the responsibility of the planner that the meal should be planned in such a way so that the requirements of all individuals are adequately met without much spending of money and energy.

OBJECTIVES OF MEAL PLANNING

- Meeting the nutritional requirement of all individuals according to their ages and activities.
- Minimizing the expenditure or spending according to the estimated food budget.
- Including the food from each food group
- To consider the family size and composition
- Considering the foods according to the choices and tastes of members
- Cooking the food in such a way so that no more nutrients are lost
- Minimizing the time and energy expenditures.

PRINCIPLES OF MEAL PLANNING

For living a healthy and prosperous life man eats food. Food taken by every organism is regarded as the source of energy and is the important factor for surviving in the community. For achieving a good health a balanced diet is needed and for making the diet balanced a careful planning of meal is required.

A well planned menu should be nutritionally adequate, acceptable, and economically feasible. Thus, the basic principles should be followed while planning the meal:

1. *Nutritional adequacy*: The diet planning should be nutritionally adequate. The planning of the meal should be done in such a way that the physical well-being of each member of the family is achieved. The meal which is planned should include the vital nutrients like proteins, carbohydrates, fats, vitamins and minerals. These nutrients should be present in a well proportionate manner. For example, the proportion of carbohydrate, fat and protein should be in the ratio of 7:1:2.

2. *Fulfilling the family needs*: In a family the members of different age and sex live together. A child living in a family requires more proteins as he/she is in the growing period. If there is an adolescent then a nutritionally adequate diet should be required. Pregnant woman needs more protein and iron rich diet and the elderly needs proteinecious and vitamin rich diet. Thus, the meal planning varies with the age, occupation and lifestyle of the family.

3. *Inclusion of food from food groups*: The inclusion of a wide variety of foods in meal planning ensures the presence of nutrients not found in some foods but abundant in others. The selection of food from all food groups, in planning meals, ensures an adequate intake of the nutrients that perform all the major functions of the body. These foods contain the nutrients like protein, carbohydrates, and fats, and the group of vitamins and minerals, which are necessary for carrying out all the physical and mental activities.

4. *Economic feasibility*: Money is the most important factor which affects the meal planning. The meal planned which is not within budget, cannot be practiced for a longer period of time. The cost of the meals can be reduced by including the seasonally available foods in preparing the meals as they are easily purchased and also contains the nutrients in good amount.

5. *Likes and dislikes of the family*: While planning meals the likes and dislikes of the members are also considered. The people have different preferences such as some are vegetarian and some prefers nonveg. If the members do not like greens, then the planning should be done for satisfying the nonvegetarian. Also the cultural, religious and traditional aspects, while planning the meal should not be neglected.

6. *Healthy considerations*: Besides nutritional adequacy, the meal should provide the bio-active components such as antioxidants. For this, the greens and fruits are the right choice for enhancing the nutritional value of the meal.

7. *Saving the time and energy*: Planning the meals requires the expenditure of time and energy. So the planning should be done in such a way that energy and time is consumed. For this the various devices and utensils should be used. The recipes planned should be simple and should be nutritious.

8. *Variety in meals*: Eating the same food daily is not preferred by anyone. The enjoyment of meal is enhanced by having different foods on each day and for this the planning of meal is done in such a way that daily different recipes are cooked keeping in mind the nutritional quality.

9. *Hygienic practices*: Maintaining hygienic practices in the surroundings helps in keeping the microorganisms away. Washing of food items and utensils removes the microorganisms and thus the health is not affected.

Points to be remembered in meal planning:

- Planning of the meals should be done in such a way that minimum RDA must be met for all nutrients.
- Two cereals should be included during meal preparation.
- The foods such as green leafy vegetables and roots and tubers must be included as they are rich in fibre and gives satiety.
- Energy derived from cereals should not be less than 75 per cent.
- The pulses should be taken 2–3 times daily. The germinated pulses are more nutritious and add variety in diet.
- The flour used for making chapati should not be sieved as this reduces the bran content which is good sources of vitamins and fibre.
- The fruit should not be peeled and should not be taken in form of juice as it results in loss of vitamin C, they should be eaten as raw.
- The meal prepared should be low in fat, saturated fats and cholesterol.
- The use of refined flour such as maida, should be minimized.
- The foods from all the food groups should be included as no single food has all the nutrients.
- Salt and sugar must be used in moderation.
- The colored foods such as vegetables and fruits should be included during meal preparation as they are good sources of antioxidants.
- Milk and milk preparations such as curd, sweets should be included as they provide

energy and curd is a good source of probiotics.

- Eggs and fishes should be taken as they are good sources of proteins and adds variety in diet.
- Water should be taken in adequate amount.
- Food exchange list must be used for calculation.
- The seasonal fruits and vegetables should be used in preparing the meal as they are cheap and nutritionally good.
- The cultural and religious aspect should also be kept in mind and the preparation should be done keeping these aspects in mind.
- The meal should not be cooked for a longer period of time.
- The meal should be cooked in a clean environment. The vegetables and fruits should be washed before consumption.
- The budget should also be kept in mind while planning the meal. The money should be spent in such a way that all the food items are well included.
- The texture and taste should be kept in mind. These make the food acceptable. For example, salad must be prepared and raita is a good way of enhancing taste with other items.

MEAL PLANNING FOR SCHOOL GOING CHILDREN

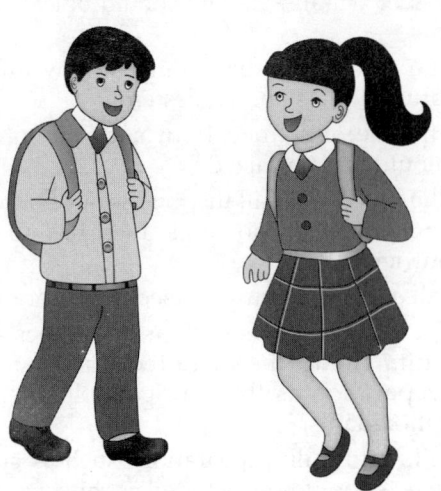

The children from the age of 7 years to 12 years are regarded as the school going children. At this stage the growth of child occurs at slower rate. During the school years the rate of further growth slows down, however, it does not mean that no significant growth is occurring. The growth occurs at a steady rate. The school age is characterized by an improvement of the muscular growth and other parts of the body. As the growth of the muscles and other tissues occurs, so nutritional requirement also increases.

As school year is regarded as the period of growth, therefore it is important that the good foundation of health is laid during this period. Thus, the important way through which the growth and development are achieved, is to supply a nutritionally balanced diet. A nutritionally balanced diet is crucial in fostering the optimum growth and development of the child.

Growth pattern (1–6 years)

At the age of 2 years, the increase in height is about 10 cm and weight gain is 2 to 2.5 kg. After two years annual gain in height and weight are only 6 to 7 cm and 1.5 to 2 kg respectively. However, a wide variation in the physical development of children is observed.

As growth proceeds, changes are observed in proportion of muscle tissue, fat deposits and skeletal structure. The body fluid gradually decreases and there are adipose tissue and bones increased due to mineralization.

At the age of 2 years psychosocial change also occurs. At this age a sense of individuality is reflected in his food behavior. As the age increases, sense of independence, initiative, imagination and curiosity also increase.

Preschool age is also regarded as a period of imitation and sex identification. The boys imitate their fathers and girls their mothers. Same behavior is reflected at meal times, they prefer the meals according to the likes and dislikes of their parents and therefore, the parents play an important role in developing healthy and positive attitude towards food.

Growth pattern (6–12 years)

The age from 6 to 12 years is the crucial, as the rate of growth is slow but adequate reserves are laid down during this period for the rapid growth during adolescence.

The girls have a less percentage of muscle tissues but they have higher deposition of body fat as compared to boys of the same age. Boys are taller and heavier than girls at each stage, but at the age of 11 to 12 years girls become heavier and taller.

As the child enters in school life, he/she develops ability to work out problems and participate in group activities. This is a period of emotional stress, competitive behavior and dreaming which brings a drastic change in the previous learning and personality pattern. There is a change from dependence of parental standards towards those set by peer group.

RDAs for school going children

As children go to school, hence they need extra energy and protein. In school the children spent his/her 5–6 hours and do various activities. At school they learn, for this they have to use their mental capacity, during their play time they need physical energy, thus the food rich in carbohydrates must be given to the child.

A protein is the most important nutrient which must be given to the child for growth of body parts and for the maintenance of the tissues. During play at home or at school the child receives various injuries and thus the diet given to the child must have the enough protein so that the worn out tissues are well repaired with the growth of new cells and tissues. The proteins are also essential for attaining the growth. For this the pulses, milk, greens and fruits must be given to the child.

For proper formation of bones and for continuous mineralization, the calcium and phosphorus must be provided in the diet. The child must be given milk and milk products such as paneer, butter, curd and cheese so that calcium is easily retained in the body. About 400 mg of calcium a child must get daily in the diet.

Iron is another mineral that is required for your child's growth and development. Having a diet with foods that are high in iron is necessary for the formation of strong muscles and hemoglobin and thus anemia is prevented among children. For having a good reserve of iron in the body, the foods such as green leafy vegetables, fish, peanut butter, nuts, and watermelon must be included in the diet of the children.

The diet of the child must also contain adequate amount of vitamins for preventing the diseases. The vitamins such as vitamin A must be given for preventing night blindness and also for maintaining the structural integrity of the cells. The other vitamins such as vitamin B are necessary for maintaining the normal functioning of body processes. Vitamin C is necessary for preventing scurvy and for healthy formation of gums and teeth. The vitamins such as vitamin D, vitamin E and vitamin K are also essential for maintenance of the body parts and tissues.

The likes and dislikes of the children vary from time to time. During their breakfast they want to have small meal while during their lunch time they demand for different things. After coming from school they want to have some spicy and tasty. Thus the meal should have a variety and the planning should be done in such a way that they don't feel bore and have their meal enthusiastically. The meal should contain various food items which should be nutritious and should fulfill the nutritional requirement of the child. Besides nutrition, the taste and appearance of the meal should also be considered.

Table 4.1: Recommended dietary allowances prescribed by ICMR

NUTRIENTS	Age (in years)	
	1–3	4–6
Energy (kcal)	1240	1690
Protein (g)	22	30
Fat (g)	25	25
Calcium (mg)	400	400
Iron (mg)	12	18
Vitamin A:		
Retinol (μg)	400	400
β-Carotene (μg)	1600	1600
Vitamin B:		
Thiamine (mg)	0.6	0.9
Riboflavin (mg)	0.7	1.0
Niacin (mg)	8	11
Vitamin C (mg)	40	40
Pyridoxine (mg)	0.9	0.9
Folic acid (μg)	30	40
Vitamin B$_{12}$ (μg)	0.2–1	2–1

Table 4.2: ICMR recommended dietary allowances of school going children age (in years)

NUTRIENTS	Age (in years)		
	7–9	10–12	
		Boys	Girls
Energy (kcal)	1950	2190	1950
Protein (gm)	41	54	57
Fat (gm)	25	22	22
Calcium (mg)	400	600	600
Iron	26	34	19
Vitamin A:			
Retinol (μg)	600	600	600
β-Carotene (μg)	2400	2400	2400
Thiamine (mg)	1.0	1.1	1.1
Riboflavin (mg)	1.2	1.3	1.2
Niacin (mg)	13	15	13
Pyridoxine (mg)	1.6	1.6	1.6
Ascorbic acid (mg)	40	40	40
Folic acid (mg)	60	70	70
Vitamin B$_{12}$ (mg)	0.2–1	0.2–1	0.2–1

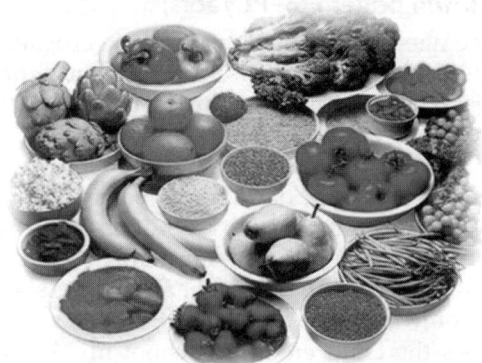

APPROACHES FOR DEVELOPING HEALTHY EATING HABITS AMONG CHILDREN

Some of the important approaches of developing healthy eating habits among children include:

• **Make healthful choices:** The choices of the food should be made from a wide variety of healthful foods which are available in the house. This practice will help the child to eat every kind of food and also a good health of the child will be laid.

• **Encouraging child to eat slowly:** The children should be asked to chew the food thoroughly and eat slowly. This will aid in digestion and constipation will not develop.

• **Encouraging the child to drink water:** Water is an important source of electrolytes and helps in maintaining the electrolyte balance in the body. Drinking water helps in digestion and also the regulation of body activities are well maintained.

• **Eating the meals with all family members:** During meal time all the members should be gathered and the eating should be proceeded with the pleasant mood and with conversations. This will help in developing the interest among the children and the children will not leave the table also, the meal will become more delicious with conversation and stress will also be removed to some extent but along with this the conversation should not be run all the time, otherwise the concentration on the meal will not drawn so much.

• **Discourage the child eating meals or snacks while watching TV.** The meal should be served only in designated areas of the home, such as the dining room. Eating in front of the TV may make it difficult to pay attention to feelings of fullness, and may lead to overeating.

- **Washing the hands before eating:** Washing of hand before eating is a good habit which helps in preventing the diseases. This is because we never know the kinds of bacteria that have been living in our hand. While eating they enters in our body and thus illness may be caused. Thus we should clean our hands thoroughly with the soap and then the food should be eaten.

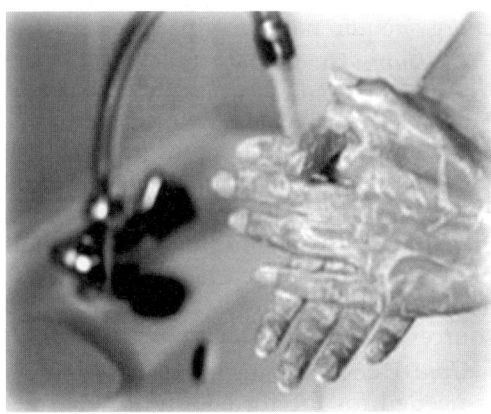

- **Avoid too much fat in the diet:** The children should be warned about the harmful effects of the fat and he/she should be discouraged from eating the more fatty foods as this may lead to obesity among the children.

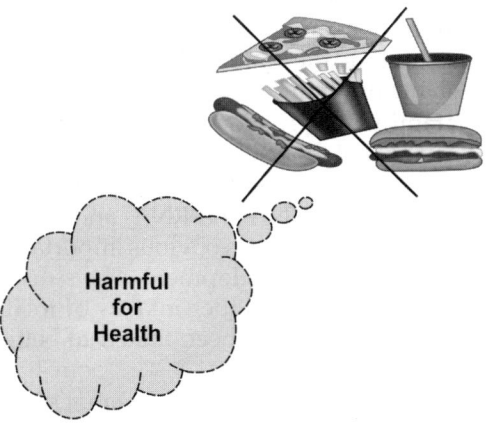

Harmful for Health

- **Aware the child from eating outside:** Children should be aware from the threats of the outside food. The food taken from outside is not nutritious and sometime it is contaminated with germs and other microorganisms. Also the food prepared is not well handled and harmful diseases may occur.

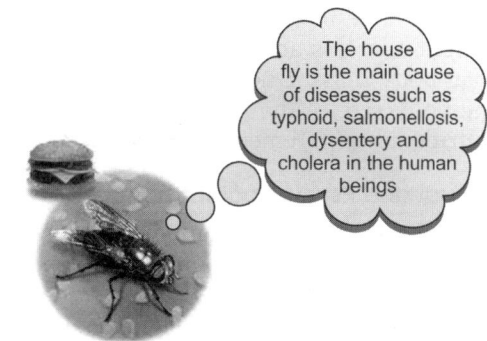

The house fly is the main cause of diseases such as typhoid, salmonellosis, dysentery and cholera in the human beings

MEAL PLANNING FOR ADOLESCENTS

Adolescence is a period between school going age and adulthood. A child between 13 and 18 years of age is called an adolescent. Adolescence is the period of rapid growth. At this period physical, physiological, and psychological developments of the children occur.

PHYSICAL, PSYCHOLOGICAL AND SOCIAL CHANGES

The final growth spurt occurs during this period. The process of physical development of a child occurs at this stage. Among girls the growth spurt occurs at approximately 11–14 years and in boys 13–16 years. The height and weight increases at maximum rate, however, after menarche the increase in the height stops. In boys growth of height and weight continues till the age of 18–20 years.

Body size

The child attains full physical development at this stage. The changes in the body size occur due to hormonal changes which regulate the development of sex characteristics.

The growth of the bones continues for a longer period of time for boys than girls. The skeleton reaches its full maturity by 17 years in the boys and among the girls the skeleton attains maturity by the age of 20. With the mineralization of the bones the water content of the body also decreases. The deposition of fat is more among the girls, whereas boys add more muscle mass. These pubertal changes lead the boys to have more lean body mass, skeletal weight and less adipose tissue as a ratio of total body mass. Due to these differences in the body size of the girls and the boys, the nutritional requirements also vary.

Sexual and Psychosocial Changes

The growth spurt is accompanied by sexual maturity which is a very important aspect of adolescence. In girls there is development of breasts, auxiliary and pubic hair and menarche and in boys the deepening of voice, broadening of shoulders, development of auxiliary and pubic hair, growth of penis and testicles, occur. As this period is a transition to adulthood, the girls and the boys try to develop self identity. They want to be accepted in their peer group along with the changes in their food habits, dressing also occur. This in turn brings psychological, emotional and social stresses due to which the nutritional needs are also affected to a great extent.

Recommended Dietary Allowances (RDAs) for Adolescents

Energy: The need of the energy increases with the growth and development. Boys belonging to the age groups of 13 to 18 need between 2450 and 2600 calories each day, whereas adolescent girls need approximately 2060 calories each day. This is a significant increase in the amount of the energy requirements. To meet these calorie needs, the diet should be chosen by including a variety of healthful foods such as whole grains, fruits, and vegetables and low-fat dairy products. The metabolic demands of growth and energy expenditure increases the calorie needs. According to the committee of Indian Council of Medical Research, the diet should be planned on the basis of ideal weight for age.

Proteins: Protein is important for growth and maintenance of muscle. Adolescents need between 60 and 70 grams of protein each day. The requirement of proteins can be easily met by intake of beef, pork, chicken, eggs and dairy products. Protein is also available from certain vegetable sources, including tofu and other soy foods, beans and nuts. The protein needs represent 12–14 percent of the total energy requirements.

Calcium: The intake of calcium is essential for development of strong and dense bones. The deficiency of calcium during adolescence and young adulthood puts individuals at risk for developing osteoporosis later in life. For preventing the bone disorders, adolescents are encouraged to consume three to four servings of calcium-rich foods each day. The foods such as milk, yogurt, cheese and curd are good sources of calcium.

Iron: Due to gain in muscle mass, more iron is needed for the formation of new muscle cells and to obtain oxygen for energy. The deficiency of iron causes anemia, which leads to fatigue, confusion, and weakness. The diet of the adolescents thus includes the foods such as beef, chicken, whole grain and green leafy vegetables.

Vitamins: The diet must contain adequate amount of vitamins for the normal functioning of the body.

- **Vitamin A** is an important vitamin for preventing the night blindness and for enhancing immunity.
- **Vitamin B$_6$** is required for carrying out various metabolic activities.
- **Folate** is required for the synthesis of nucleic acids (DNA and RNA) and amino acids. Thus, folate has obvious importance in growth and development. The studies have shown that higher intakes of folate in adolescents have been linked to better academic achievement.
- **Vitamin B$_{12}$** is needed for metabolism of proteins and lipids. The deficiency of vitamin B$_{12}$ causes the damaging of the

myelin sheath covering cranial, spinal and peripheral nerves, resulting in neurological damage. The myelin sheath is the insulating layer of tissue made up of lipids and proteins that surrounds nerve fibres and also helps in allowing rapid and efficient transmission of nerve impulses. In some cases, neurologic symptoms caused by vitamin B_{12} deficiency can be reversed by vitamin treatment, but reversibility seems to be dependent upon the duration of the associated neurologic complications. Vitamin B_{12} is naturally present only in animal products, such as meat, poultry, fish (including shellfish), and to a lesser extent in milk.

- **Vitamin C** is required for the synthesis of collagen, carnitine and neurotransmitters. Vitamin C is also a highly effective antioxidant and is important for enhancing immunity. Vitamin C also enhances the absorption of non-heme iron by reducing dietary ferric iron (Fe^{3+}) to ferrous iron (Fe^{2+}).

- **Vitamin D** is another important vitamin needed for the proper maintaining normal calcium metabolism and is therefore, necessary for bone health. Severe vitamin D deficiency results in the failure of bone to mineralize and may lead to rickets and osteoporosis. Rapidly growing bones are most severely affected by rickets. Food and Nutrition Noard (FNB), 2010, of the institute of medicine set RDA for vitamin D—600 IU/day (15 mcg/day) for adolescents aged 14 to 18 years.

Table 4.3: ICMR recommended dietary allowances for adolescents

Nutrients	Boys		Girls	
	13–15 yrs	16–18 yrs	13–15 yrs	16–18 yrs
Energy (kcal)	2450	2640	2060	2060
Protein (g)	70	78	65	63
Fat (g)	22	22	22	22
Calcium (mg)	600	500	600	500
Iron (mg)	41	50	28	30

Contd.

Table 4.3: ICMR recommended dietary allowances for adolescents *(Contd.)*

Nutrients	Boys		Girls	
	13–15 yrs	16–18 yrs	13–15 yrs	16–18 yrs
Vitamin A				
Retinol (mg)	600	600	600	600
β-Carotene (μg)	2400	2400	2400	2400
Thiamine (mg)	1.2	1.3	1.0	1.0
Riboflavin (mg)	1.5	1.6	1.2	1.2
Niacin (mg)	16	17	14	14
Pyridoxine (mg)	2.0	2.0	2.0	2.0
Vitamin C (mg)	40	40	40	40
Folic acid (mg)	100	100	100	100
Vitamin B_{12} (mg)	0.2–1.0	0.2–1.0	0.2–1.0	0.2–1.0

Points to be considered while planning meals for adolescents

The meal planning for adolescent is a complex task due to the variation in mood and the age groups. The planning of the meal should be made on the basis of their age groups, besides this the other factors such as nutritional value of the food, acceptability and availability of food, etc. should also be considered. It is also necessary to know the routine and gender of the children. Based on these criteria, following facts should be kept in mind while planning the meal for adolescents:

1. The foods from each food group should be included in the diet.

2. While preparing the food, mixture of cereals and pulses should be used so that the quality of protein is enhanced. Animal protein can also be added, if possible and acceptable.

3. The fluids should be included in sufficient quantity.

4. Too much fat should not be used while preparing food as it may lead to pimples and stomach disorders.

5. The meal should be taken at regular intervals of time.

6. The weight should be checked regularly. If one is underweight, the amount of calories in diet should be increased and if one is overweight, the intake of fat should be reduced.

7. The fibrous foods like vegetables, fruits, salad, *etc.* are good sources of antioxidants and should be included.

Dietary Guidelines

Psychological pressures on adolescents influence their eating habits. Boys generally tend to have a better appetite than girls and this helps them to meet their nutritional demands. Hence, adolescents should consume a balanced diet including iron, calcium, protein, mineral and vitamins rich foods. They should avoid junk foods as they provide empty calories and are not nutritious. They should not miss their meals and during meal time the emotions and tensions should be kept away and attention should be drawn only on food.

MEAL PLANNING FOR ADULTS

Adulthood is another crucial period of human life. The adulthood is regarded as the period of strength, enthusiasm, activity and responsibility for both men and women. Men have the responsibility of earning for the family, to feed them and to fulfill the needs of

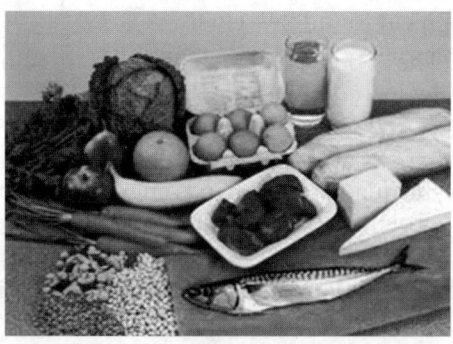

the members of the family and women have the responsibility to look after the husband and her children, for this she has to carry out the various activities at home as well as at outside. Thus for doing the duties well the health of both man and woman should be good and for this, optimal nutrition is essential for maintaining the health.

During adulthood, body growth and height stop to a certain extent, but tissue breakdown and repairing of body tissues continues. Therefore, adequate amount of essential nutrients are needed for maintenance of physical and mental healths in adults.

Recommended Dietary Allowances (RDAs) for Adults

Energy: The requirement of energy is based on the reference man and woman (explained earlier). The energy needs of adults depend on the physical activity they do. The energy needs are high for those whose occupation entails heavy work, however, the allowances will be less for those who are involved in the sedentary or moderate work. The RDAs are shown in Table 4.4 as suggested by ICMR.

Proteins: Studies on Indian adults have revealed that the minimum intake of dietary protein to maintain nitrogen equilibrium, on an average, is 0.58 g/kg body weight. After allowing for sweat losses the intake works out to 0.7 g/kg. The corresponding safe level of intake has been computed to be 0.88 g/kg body weight. Hence, the ICMR has recommended 1.0 g protein per kg body weight for both men and women. Since protein needs are not affected by activity, the RDA for a protein is 60 g/day and 50 g/day for adult man and adult woman respectively.

Fat: About 20% of the energy is derived from fats. The invisible fat provides 9% of energy while the visible fat provides 10%. Thus, about 10–20 g of fat should be provided daily in the diet.

About 12 g of visible fat provides 3% of linoleic acid of the total energy requirement. To provide energy density and palatability to the diet, the ICMR has suggested 20 g visible fat per day. A high amount of saturated fatty acids is present in the oils may increase the linoleic acid requirements and are detrimental to health. Hence, ICMR recommends that the combination of oils should be equal with equal proportion of saturated, monounsaturated and polyunsaturated fatty acids.

Minerals

Calcium and phosphorus: Calcium is important for replacing calcium lost from body through urine, faeces, sweat and bile. For these activities positive calcium balance needs to be maintained and this can be achieved by an intake of 300 to 500 mg of calcium daily. ICMR has suggested 400 mg calcium/day for both men and women.

A desirable intake of phosphorus is recommended, with the intake of calcium, as the functions of calcium and phosphorus are necessary for mineralization of bones. It is suggested that the ratio of calcium and phosphorus should remain 1:1 and during infancy the suggested Ca:P ratio is 1:1.5.

Iron: Women needs additional iron due to loss of iron during menstruation which varies between 0.5 and 1 mg per day. For meeting the iron requirements the women needs 30 mg per day and men requires only 28 mg per day.

Vitamins: Vitamins are necessary for the normal functioning of tissues and other body organs. The requirement of vitamins varies with the activities and age of the adults.

Table 4.4: ICMR recommended dietary allowances for adults

Sex	Activity	Energy (kcal)	Protein (g)	Fat (g)	Calcium (g)	Iron (mg)	Vitamin A		Thiamine (mg)	Riboflavin (mg)	Niacin (mg)	Pyridoxin (mg)	Vit.C (mg)	Vit. B_{12} (μg)
							Retinol (μg)	β-Carotene (μg)						
M A L E S	Sedentary	2425	60	20	400	28	600	2400	1.2	1.4	16	2.0	40	1
	Moderate	2845	60	20	400	28	600	2400	1.4	1.6	18	2.0	40	1
	Heavy	3800	60	20	400	28	600	2400	1.6	1.9	21	2.0	40	1
F E M A L E S	Sedentary	1875	60	20	400	30	600	2400	6.0	1.1	12	2.0	40	1
	Moderate	2225	60	20	400	30	600	2400	1.1	1.3	14	2.0	40	1
	Heavy	2925	60	20	400	30	600	2400	1.2	1.5	16	2.0	40	1

Points to be considered while planning meals for adults:

- The balanced diet should comprise enough fibre, pulses, whole grains, fresh fruits and vegetables.
- The foods containing oil or sugar should be avoided as these increase the cholesterol level and calorie intake in the body.
- Excessive salt should be avoided.
- The processed foods containing high calories, saturated fats, added sugar, refined cereal grains, and artificial additives should not be consumed.
- Carbonated drinks should not be taken.
- Exercise should be taken daily.
- The foods that are rich in certain minerals like calcium, iron and iodine should be taken daily especially by women.
- The intake of alcohol should be limited and smoking should be avoided.
- Ample amounts of water and fluid should be taken at regular interval of time for proper digestion of foods.

BALANCED DIET FOR ADULTS AS SUGGESTED BY NATIONAL INSTITUTE OF NUTRITION (NIN), HYDERABAD

Table 4.5: Sample menu for adult man (sedentary)

Meal time	Food group	Raw amounts	Cooked recipe	Servings
BREAKFAST	Milk	100 ml	Milk or	½ Cup
	Sugar	15 g	Tea or	2 Cups
			Coffee	1 Cup
	Cereals	70 g	Breakfast item	
	Pulses	20 g		
LUNCH	Cereals	150 g	Rice	2 Cups
			Phulkas	2 Nos.
	Vegetables	150 g	Veg. curry	¾ Cup
	Pulses	20 g	Dhal	½ Cup
	Vegetables	50 gm	Veg. salad	7–8 Slices
	Milk	100 ml	Curd	½ Cup
TEA	Cereals	50 g	Snack	
	Milk	50 ml	Tea	1 Cup
	Sugar	10 g		
DINNER	Cereals	150 g	Rice	2 Cups
			Phulkas	2 Nos.
	Vegetables	150 g	Veg. curry	¾ Cups
	Pulses	20 g	Dhal	½ Cups
	Vegetables	50 g	Veg. raita	
	Milk(curd)	50 ml		½ Cup
	Fruit	100 g	Seasonal	1 Medium

1 Cup = 200 ml

Note: For non-vegetarians – substitute one pulse portion with one portion of egg/meat/chicken/fish.

Breakfast Items: Idli — 4 Nos./Dosa — 3 Nos./Upma — 1–1/2 cup/Bread — 4 Slices/Porridge — 2 Cups/Cornflakes with milk — 2 Cups.

Snacks: Poha — 1 Cup/Toast — 2 Slices/Samosa — 2/Sandwiches — 2/Biscuits — 5

Table 4.6: Sample menu for adult woman (sedentary)

Meal time	Food group	Raw amounts	Cooked recipe	Servings
BREAKFAST	Milk	100 ml	Milk or	½ Cup
	Sugar	15 g	Tea or	2 Cups
			Coffee	1 Cup
	Cereals	50 g	Breakfast item	
	Pulses	20 g		
LUNCH	Cereals	100 g	Rice	1 Cup
			Phulkas	2 Nos.
	Vegetables	100 g	Veg. curry	½ Cup
	Pulses	20 g	Dhal	½ Cup
TEA	Cereals	50 g	Snack	
	Milk	50 ml	Tea	1 Cup
	Sugar	10 g		

Contd.

Table 4.6: Sample menu for adult woman (sedentary) *(Contd.)*

Meal time	Food group	Raw amounts	Cooked recipe	Servings
	Cereals	100 g	Rice	1 Cup
			Phulkas	2 Nos.
DINNER	Vegetables	100 g	Veg. curry	½ Cup
	Pulses	20 g	Dhal	½ Cup
	Vegetables	50 g	Veg. raita	
	Milk(Curd)	50 ml		½ Cup
	Fruit	100 g	Seasonal	1 Medium

1 Cup = 200 ml

Note: For nonvegetarians — Substitute one pulse portion with one portion of egg/meat/chicken/fish.

Use 20 g visible fat per day.

Breakfast Items: Idli — 4 Nos./Dosa — 2 Nos./Upma — 1 Cup/Bread — 3 Slices/Porridge — 1/2–1 Cups/Cornflakes with milk — 1/2–1 Cups.

Snacks: Poha — 1 Cup/ Toast — 2 Slices/Samosa — 2/Sandwiches — 2/Biscuits — 5

MEAL PLANNING DURING PREGNANCY

Pregnancy is the most beautiful period of a woman's life. This is a period of great physiological as well as psychological stress for the women. The period of pregnancy is regarded as the period of great concern as the mother has to maintain her optimum health and also she has to prepare for delivery and also for the period of lactation. She has to take good nutrition for the development of the foetus and also for her health. Adequate nutrition before and during pregnancy is very important for a long-term health. A woman who has been well nourished before conception can fulfill the needs of the growing foetus, so that good health of the baby is laid and good health is enjoyed till entire lifespan. For laying the good health of the child, mother's diet should contain adequate nutrients which are necessary for the normal well-being of the child and also the maternal stores do not get depleted and produce sufficient milk to nourish her child after birth.

The mothers who are undernourished, give birth to the children who are at an increased risk of being premature, or born with low birth weight and are malformed. Intrauterine nutrition is highly important for the growth and development of the foetus.

Physiological changes in pregnancy

The physiological changes such as increase in blood sugar and cardiac output occur during pregnancy. Some other changes observed are as follows:

The changes in the hormones occur during this time. Levels of progesterone and estrogens rise continually throughout pregnancy and menstrual cycle is suppressed. The hormone estrogen is produced by the placenta which is associated for providing nourishment for fetal well-being. There also occurs an increment in the levels of human chorionic gonadotropin, produced by the placenta. This hormone is also responsible for maintaining the level of progesterone produced by the corpus luteum. The increased progesterone produced, later by the placenta, helps in relaxation of smooth muscle.

The levels of prolactin are also increased which bring a change in the structure of the mammary gland from ductal to lobular-alveolar. The levels of parathyroid hormone is also increased which helps in increasing the calcium uptake in the gut and reabsorption by the kidney. With these hormones the level of cortical and aldosterone are also increased. The human placental lactogen hormone produced by placenta stimulates lipolysis and fatty acid metabolism by the women and conserving blood glucose for use by the fetus.

During pregnancy the structure of the body size changes with a rapid rate. During the first three months of the pregnancy about 1.5 kg of weight is gained which is accompanied by excessive vomiting. Excessive vomiting can cause a slight loss of weight gain. In each subsequent months the average gain should be 1.5 kg being a little more in the last two months. At full term the total gain is about 10–12 kg. The sudden gains or losses may be harmful.

The level of the blood volume increases by 50% which is required to carry nutrients to the fetus via the blood stream and removing the metabolic waste from the fetus. With increase in blood volume, the concentration of plasma proteins, hemoglobin, blood glucose and water soluble vitamins decrease. The decline in serum albumin level tends to accumulate extracellular water during pregnancy. The level of hemoglobin also changes and it drops to 11 g/100 ml (normal range 12–13 g/100 ml) despite an increase in total hemoglobin content. Thus, the women with hemoglobin levels less than 10 g/100 ml are considered anemic, during pregnancy.

Recommended Dietary Allowances For Pregnant Women

Energy: During pregnancy the caloric requirements are increased for maintaining the growth of the fetus, placenta and maternal tissues and for the increased basal metabolic rate. At the initial stage of the pregnancy the caloric requirements are minimal but the demands increase sharply towards the end of the first trimester and during the second and third trimesters, the energy requirement becomes constant. The energy requirement for a moderately active adult woman is about 40 kcal/kg body weight. Indian Council of Medical Research nutrition expert group, 2010, has suggested additional 350 kcal per day during the period of pregnancy. The foods such as rice, wheat, bajra, ragi, jowar and roots and tubers should be considered during pregnancy for fulfilling the energy requirement.

Protein: The protein demand is also increased in the second half of pregnancy. During pregnancy the Indian Council of Medical Research, (2010), recommend an additional 23 g/day of protein. The additional protein is essential to meet growing demands of increasing tissues.

Fats: Therefore an intake of 30 g of visible fat has been suggested to meet the essential fatty acid needs.

MINERALS

Calcium: The calcium requirement for an adult woman is 400 mg/day. During pregnancy the need increases to 1200 mg/day. The additional calcium is needed for the growth and development of bones as well as teeth of the fetus and also for the protection of calcium resources of the mother to meet the high demand of calcium during lactation.

Iron: The requirement of iron increases from 30 mg/day to 35 mg/day during pregnancy. The iron is needed for the expansion of maternal tissues including red cell mass, iron content of placenta and blood loss during parturition. Iron also helps in building the iron store in fetal liver to last for at least 4–6 months after birth. The infants are born with extra reserve of iron, 18–22 g/100 ml.

Other minerals: Iodine, zinc and sodium are required for reducing the complications of pregnancy and for increasing the extracellular fluid.

Vitamins: A good intake of all vitamins is essential at the time of pregnancy. Vitamin D is required for reducing muscular cramps of pregnancy and also for maternal calcium absorption and for calcium metabolism of infant. Vitamin E is necessary for preventing abortions and vitamin K is needed for preventing neonatal hemorrhages. Vitamin B_6 or folic acid is very important to prevent macrocytic anaemia and promote normal fetal growth, as it prevents serious birth defects.

Fibres: The diet should contain the fibre rich foods to prevent constipation. The foods such as whole fruits and vegetables, whole grain cereals, vegetable soups and whole pulses are good sources of fibres.

Water: For keeping the body hydrated, for preventing constipation, hemorrhoids, and for flushing out the toxins, water should be taken at regular intervals of time.

Table 4.7: ICMR recommended dietary allowances for an expectant mother

Nutrient	Normal adult woman	Pregnant woman
Energy (kcal)		
Sedentary	1875	2175
Moderate	2225	2525
Heavy	2925	3225
Protein (g)	50	65
Fat (g)	20	30
Calcium (mg)	400	1000
Iron (mg)	30	38
Vitamin A		
Retinol (µg)	600	600
(or)		
β-Carotene (µg)	2400	2400
Thiamine (mg)		
Sedentary	0.9	1.1
Moderate	1.1	1.3
Heavy	1.2	1.4
Riboflavin (mg)		
Sedentary	1.1	1.3
Moderate	1.3	1.5
Heavy	1.5	1.7
Niacin (mg)		
Sedentary	12	14
Moderate	14	16
Heavy	16	18
Pyridoxine (mg)	2.0	2.5
Ascorbic acid (mg)	40	40
Folic acid (mg)	100	400
Vitamin B_{12} (mg)	1	1

Points to be considered while planning meal during pregnancy

A good, healthy and nutritious diet taken during pregnancy helps in laying the foundation of good health of the baby during the whole period of life. While planning meal for expectant mothers, following points should be kept in mind:

1. The foods rich in fats like nuts, seeds such as flaxseeds, dairy products like paneer and avocados should be included in the diet.
2. The foods which are rich sources of vitamins like guava, mango, tomatoes, grapefruit, papaya and watermelon, amaranth, broccoli, sprouts, spinach, sweet potato, carrots should be included while planning meals.
3. The food items such as milk and dairy products, green leafy vegetables, and fortified foods; iron found in leafy vegetables, fruits like apple and guava, nuts and seeds, should be taken daily.
4. During pregnancy constipation is a common problem thus the foods rich in fibre content should be included during meal planning.
5. The women should take a well balanced diet during pregnancy.
6. The foods from all the food groups should be included.
7. The diet during pregnancy has to be rich in calories, proteins, vitamins and minerals and balanced.

STUDY QUESTIONS

1. What do you mean by meal planning? What principles are involved in meal planning?
2. What is the necessity of developing good food habits among the school going children? What points are considered while planning meals for the school going children?
3. What are the physical, psychological and social changes occur during adolescence? What is the importance of good nutrition during adolescence?
4. What points are considered while planning meals for adult women? Give balanced diet for sedentary women.
5. Why pregnancy is considered as the crucial period of life? Plan a meal for pregnant women.

5 Nutrients and their Functions

Nutrients are the constituents in food that are supplied to the body in suitable amounts. These are the essential chemicals that an organism needs to live and grow. These are the substances which are involved in organism's metabolism which must be taken in form of food. Nutrients help to build and repair tissues, regulate body processes and are converted to and used as energy.

Classification of Nutrients

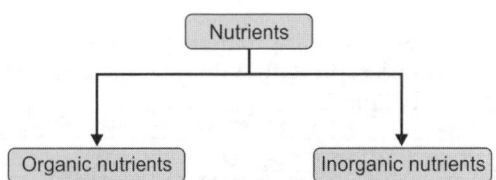

Organic nutrients: The organic nutrients include carbohydrates, fats, proteins (or their building blocks, amino acids), and vitamins.

Inorganic nutrients: These include dietary minerals and water.

Another Classification of Nutrients

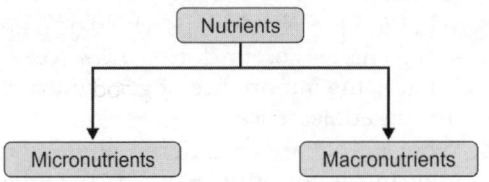

Micronutrients: The nutrients that are needed in very small amount are micronutrients. These include vitamins and minerals.

Macronutrients: The nutrients that are needed in larger quantities are called macronutrients. These include proteins, fats and carbohydrates.

How Nutrients Work in the Body

The foods we eat contain various nutrients such as carbohydrates, proteins, fats, vitamins and minerals. These nutrients from food are absorbed by the body as it passes through the digestive system. The main functions of nutrients perform in the body are:

- Nutrients are essential for growth, maintenance and repairment of the cell.
- Nutrients provide energy to enable the body to function efficiently.
- Nutrients are good sources of fibre and water.

These nutrients do not work alone in the body and are dependent on each other for carrying out the activities of the body well. The main nutrients are the macronutrients, carbohydrates, proteins, and fats and the micronutrients, vitamins and minerals.

Functions of Micronutrients

The micronutrients, vitamins and minerals help in regulation of the activities of the body. They activate enzymes, which are proteins that act as catalysts to speed up biological reactions that take place in the body.

Minerals help in formation of bones and teeth. They are essential for maintaining the water balance and for carrying out the chemical processes in the body.

Functions of macronutrients

Macronutrients help in:

- Breaking down of carbohydrates and fats, so that energy is provided to the body.
- Absorption of protein, which acts as the building blocks, necessary for cell growth and repair.

FUNCTIONS OF NUTRIENTS

Carbohydrates

Carbohydrates are the important sources of energy. Carbohydrates are the organic compounds containing the carbon, hydrogen and oxygen generally in proportion of 1:2:1. These are sugars that can be hydrolyzed to simple sugars by the action of digestive enzymes or by heating with dilute acids.

These are very important for the living organisms, serving as skeletal structures in plants and also in insects and crustaceans. These carbohydrates also occurred as food reserves in the storage organs of plants in the liver and muscles of animals. In addition, these are an important sources of energy required for the various metabolic activities of the living organisms; the energy being derived as a result of oxidation. Carbohydrates act as a lubrication agent for skeletal joints, to provide adhesion between the cells.

Classification of Carbohydrates

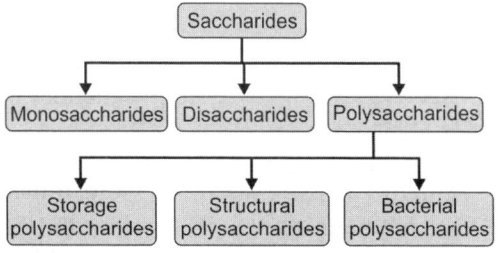

Saccharides: Saccharides are the sugars or starches, which consists of two basic compounds— the first compound is aldehyde which is composed of double-bonded carbon and oxygen atoms and an additional hydrogen atom. The other compound is ketone which is composed of double-bonded carbon and oxygen atoms, plus two additional carbon atoms.

There are three types of saccharides:

1. *Monosaccharide:* Monosaccharides are called simple sugars, consist of a single polyhydroxy aldehyde or ketone unit. The most abundant monosaccharide includes glucose, galactose or fructose. Glucose is also called dextrose, is a major source of energy for a cell and it is found in grape sugar, sweet fruits and oranges. Galactose is present in milk and dairy products, while fructose is found mostly in vegetables and fruit.

2. *Disaccharide:* Disaccharides consist of two monosaccharides joined by a glycosidic linkage. The most common disaccharides include lactose, maltose, and sucrose. If one molecule of glucose is bonded with a fructose molecule, then sucrose will be obtained, similarly lactose will be obtained, if one molecule of glucose is bonded with galactose. Sucrose is present in table sugar, molasses, beet sugar and maple sugar. Some fruits also contain sucrose. Milk is a good source of lactose.

3. *Polysaccharide:* When two or more monosaccharides are joined together they results in the formation of polysaccharides. Polysaccharide molecule chains may be made up of hundreds or thousands of monosaccharides. The chain may be branched (molecule is like a tree with branches and twigs) or unbranched (molecule is a straight line with no twigs). There are three main types of polysaccharides:

   i. **Storage polysaccharides:** Polysaccharides may act as food stores in plants in the form of starch, or food stores in humans and other animals in the form of glycogen.
      - **Glycogen:** Glycogen is the storage form of glucose in animals and humans. Glycogen is synthesized and stored mainly in the liver and

the muscles. Small amount of glycogens is found in the kidneys, and even smaller amount in certain glial cells in the brain and white blood cells. Glycogen is basically the energy reservoir in animals and humans.

- **Starch:** Starch is composed of glucose units that occur widely in plant tissues in the form of storage granules, consisting of amylose and amylopectin. Amylose molecule chains are linear (long but no branches) while amylopectin molecules are long and branch out—some amylopectin molecules are made of several thousands of glucose units. Starches are not water soluble. Starches are found chiefly in seeds, fruits, tubers, roots and stem pith of plants, notably in corn, potatoes, wheat, and rice. Humans and animals digest them by hydrolysis — our bodies have amylases which break them down. Rich sources of starches for humans include potatoes, rice and wheat.

ii. **Structural polysaccharides:** Polysaccharides also play structural roles in the plant cell wall in the form of cellulose or pectin, and the tough outer skeleton of insects in the form of chitin.

- **Cellulose:** Cellulose is an important polysaccharide. Cellulose is found in large amounts in nearly all plants, and is potentially a major source of dietary fibre. It is a non-digestible carbohydrate for humans and adds bulk to the stool. By this action it reduces chance of many gastrointestinal diseases. It also slows down digestion in your stomach and gives a feeling of satiety.

- **Chitin:** Chitin is one of the most abundant polysaccharide present in natural materials in the world. Microorganisms, such as bacteria and fungi secrete chitinases, which over time can break down into chitin.

They do not play any role in human beings.

iii. **Bacterial polysaccharides:** These are polysaccharides that are found in bacteria, especially in bacterial capsules. Pathogenic (illness causing) bacteria often produce a thick layer of mucous— like polysaccharide which cloaks the bacteria from the host's immune system. In other words, if the bacteria were in a human, that human's immune system would less likely attack the bacteria because the polysaccharide layer masks its pathogenic properties. *E. coli*, which can sometimes cause disease, produces hundreds of different polysaccharides.

Functions of Carbohydrates

Carbohydrates have a variety of functions in the animal organism; the most important is to supply energy for the body functions. Even though fat yields more energy per unit body weight than carbohydrate (9 calories per gram, as compared to 4 calories per gram), the intake of carbohydrate is greater than fat in the normal diet. The important functions of carbohydrates are as follows:

1. *Carbohydrates are the major source of energy*: Carbohydrates provide about 50–80% energy to carry out the work efficiently. Some of the carbohydrates are immediately utilized by the tissues and the remaining is stored as glycogen in the liver and muscles and some are stored as adipose tissues for future energy needs.

2. *Protein-sparing action*: If the diet lacks the calories, the most of the energy requirement is fulfilled by proteins and thus the tissue protein are broken down for maintaining the energy level. Hence, carbohydrates are mainly utilized by the body for fulfilling the major part of the energy needs, thus sparing protein for tissue building and repairing. The first physiological demand of the body is the need for energy, which must be satisfied before the nutrients are used for other functions. So, this function of

carbohydrates to spare protein for its primary purpose of body building and repair of tissues is important.

3. *Carbohydrates are essential for oxidation of fats*: Fats are also good sources of energy as carbohydrate. Besides providing energy, carbohydrates are essential for oxidation of fats. In absence of carbohydrates, fats cannot be oxidised by the body to yield energy. In the oxidation of fats oxalacetic acid, a breakdown product of carbohydrate is essential for the oxidation of acetate, which is the breakdown product of fats. In the absence of oxaloacetic acid, acetate is converted into ketone bodies, which gets accumulated in the body and the person suffers from 'Ketosis' — a toxic condition of the body. Ketosis occurs in diabetes, where the cells cannot utilize carbohydrates and in starvation, where the cells must use fat stores in the body as a source of energy.

4. *Carbohydrates play an important role in gastrointestinal function*: The lactose released from the breakdown of carbohydrates ensures and promotes the growth of a particular type of bacteria in the intestine that aids in the free flow of B complex vitamins. Lactose also helps in enhancing the absorption of calcium.

5. *Carbohydrates are important dietary fibre*: The important fibre presents in carbohydrates is cellulose adds bulk to the diet and helps in the stimulation of the peristaltic movements and secretion of important digestive enzymes.

Sources of Carbohydrates

Starchy vegetables
These include potatoes, yams, banana squashes, pumpkin, carrots, cauliflower, and beets.

Cereal grains: These include all cereals (whole or refined), such as wheat, rye, barley, rice, millet, maize and oats.

Legumes: These include peanuts, lentils, peas and beans.

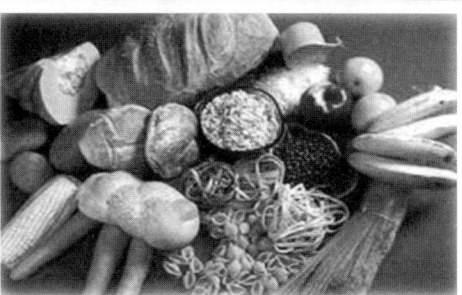

PROTEINS

Proteins are the organic compounds containing carbon, hydrogen, oxygen and nitrogen atoms. These atoms mix up in different patterns to make different amino acids which combines to form proteins by means of peptide bond, which joins a carboxylic carbon of one amino acid with nitrogen to another. The resulting peptide has a free carboxyl at one end and a free amino group at the other, permitting addition of other amino acids at the other end. Some proteins are essential because they cannot be made by the body and must be taken in diet while the others are non-essential as can be made by the liver if all the necessary chemical components are available.

Types of Proteins

Simple Proteins

The proteins yield only amino acids on hydrolysis. Some of the important simple proteins are as follows:

1. **Albumins:** These are found in plant and animal tissues and are soluble in water and dilute salt solution. These are precipitated by saturation with ammonium sulfate solution and easily coagulated by heat. These are present in blood (serum albumin), milk (lactalbumin), egg white (ovolbumin), lentils (legumelin), kidney beans (phaseolin) and wheat (leucosin).

2. **Globulins:** Globular proteins are sparingly soluble in water, soluble in neutral solutions and precipitated by dilute ammonium sulfate and coagulated by heat. These are distributed in both plant and animal tissues. These are present in

blood (serum globulins), muscle (myosin), potato (tuberin) and lentils (legumin).

3. **Glutelins:** These proteins are soluble in dilute acids and are insoluble in water and dilute salt solutions. They are found in wheat (glutenin) and rice (oryzenin).

4. **Prolamines:** Insoluble in water and absolute alcohol, soluble in 70% alcohol. These are present in wheat and rye (gliadin), corn (zein), rye (secaline) and barley (hordein).

5. **Protamines:** Soluble in water, not coagulated by heat, strongly basic, high in arginine, associate with DNA, and present in sperm cells.

6. **Histones:** Histones are soluble in water, salt solutions, and dilute acids and insoluble in ammonium hydroxide. Histone yields large amount of lysine and arginine when combined with nucleic acids within cells. They are present in thymus gland and pancreas.

7. **Scleroproteins:** These are fibrous proteins which are insoluble in all solvents and resistant to digestion. These are found in connective tissues and hard tissues. They are of three types:

   a. *Collagen:* Present in connective tissues, bones, cartilage and gelatin.

   b. *Elastin:* Ligaments, tendons and arteries contain elastin proteins.

   c. *Keratin:* Hair, nails, hooves, horns and feathers contain keratin.

Conjugated Proteins

1. **Nucleoproteins:** These are found in the cytoplasm of cells (ribonucleoprotein), nucleus of chromosomes (deoxyribonucleoprotein) viruses and bacteriophages. Nucleoproteins consist of nucleic acids, nitrogen and phosphorus. These are also present in chromosomes and in all living forms as a combination of protein with either RNA or DNA.

2. **Mucoproteins:** These proteins combined with amino sugars, sugar acids, and sulfates. These are also present in saliva (mucin) and egg white (ovomucoid).

3. **Glycoproteins:** These are present in bone (osseomucoid), tendons (tendomucoid) and carilage (chondromucoid).

4. **Phosphoproteins:** Phosphoric acid when joins with ester linkage to protein. These are found in milk (casein) and egg yolk (ovovitellin).

5. **Chromoproteins:** Hemoglobin, myoglobin, flavoproteins, respiratory pigments and cytochromes contains chromoproteins.

6. **Lipoproteins:** These are water-soluble proteins conjugated with lipids, found dispersed widely in all cells and all living forms serum lipoprotein. The brain, nerve tissues, milk and eggs contain lipoproteins.

7. **Metallo proteins:** Ferritin, carbonic anhydrase, ceruloplasmin contains metallo proteins.

Derived Proteins

1. **Proteans:** Edestan (from elastin) and myosan (from myosin) contain proteans.

2. **Proteases:** Proteases are the intermediate products of protein digestion. These are soluble in water, uncoagulated by heat, and precipitated by saturated ammonium sulfate. These are formed from partial digestion of protein by pepsin or trypsin.

3. **Peptones:** Peptones are intermediate products of protein digestion.

4. **Peptides:** The peptides are also the intermediate products of protein digestion. Two or more amino acids joined by a peptide linkage, hydrolyzed to individual amino acids.

Functions of Proteins

Proteins are very important molecules in our cells. The proteins are involved in virtually all cell functions of the body. Some proteins are involved in structural support, while others are involved in bodily movement, or in defense against germs. Proteins are constructed from a set of 20 amino acids and play important role in various life processes. The important functions of proteins are as follows:

- **Body building:** Proteins provide amino acids needed for the formation of new cells. The amino acids are supplied by food helps in formation of new tissues.
- **Defense mechanism:** Proteins helps in defending the body from antigens (foreign invaders) as they are present in antibodies which travel through the blood stream and are utilized by the immune system to identify and defend against bacteria, viruses and other foreign intruders. The antibodies destroy antigens, immobilizing them, so that they can be destroyed by white blood cells.
- **Movement of muscles:** Proteins play an important role in the movement and contraction of the muscles. The contractile proteins include actin and myosin.
- **Enzymes:** Enzymes are the catalysts that facilitate biochemical reactions. Certain enzymes are synthesized by proteins. Enzymes speed up chemical reactions and play important role in metabolic processes in the body. Enzymes like lactase break down the sugar lactose found in milk while pepsin is a digestive enzyme that helps in breaking down of proteins, present in the stomach.
- **Regulatory functions:** Hormones are messengers which help to coordinate certain bodily activities. The hormones are synthesized from the proteins. Insulin, oxytocin and somatotropin are the hormones which play important role in the body. Insulin regulates glucose metabolism by controlling the blood-sugar concentration.

Oxytocin stimulates contractions of uterus muscles in females during childbirth. Somatotropin is a growth hormone that stimulates protein production in muscle cells.

- **Structural support:** Structural proteins are fibrous and stringy and provide support. These help in the formation of the keratin, collagen and elastin. Keratins strengthen protective coverings such as hair, quills, feathers, horns and beaks. Collagens and elastin provide support for connective tissues such as tendons and ligaments.
- **Transportation:** Proteins act as carrier which moves molecules from one place to another around the body. These include hemoglobin and cytochromes. Hemoglobin transports oxygen through the blood and cytochromes operate in the electron transport chain as electron carrier proteins.
- **Gives energy:** Proteins also provides energy. A great amount of energy is provided by the metabolism of the proteins. Each gram of proteins provides about 4 kilo calories in the body.
- **Maintenance of tissues:** Proteins help in maintenance of the tissues. The proteins in the body tissues are not static and continuously broken down and replaced by new proteins synthesized from amino acids.

Sources of Proteins

Cereals, pulses, green leafy vegetables, milk, curds and fruits are good sources of proteins. Below the table is showing various foods with their protein content:

Table 5.1: Foods with their protein content

Food	Amount	Protein (gm)	Protein (gm/100 cal)
Soyabeans, cooked	1 Cup	29	1.6
Lentils, cooked	1 Cup	18	7.8
Kidney beans, cooked	1 Cup	13	6.4
Veggie burger	1 Patty	13	13.0
Peanut butter	2 Tbsp	8	4.3
Almonds	1/4 Cup	8	3.7
Soya milk, commercial, plain	1 Cup	7	7.0
Soya yogurt, plain	6 Ounces	6	4.0

Contd.

Table 5.1: Foods with their protein content *(Contd.)*

Food	Amount	Protein (gm)	Protein (gm/100 cal)
Sunflower seeds	1/4 Cup	6	3.3
Whole wheat bread	2 Slices	5	3.9
Cashews	1/4 Cup	5	2.7
Brown rice, cooked	1 Cup	5	2.1
Spinach, cooked	1 Cup	5	13.0
Potato	1 Medium	4	2.7

Sources: USDA nutrient database for standard reference, release 18, 2005 and manufacturers' information.

FATS

Fats are the essential part of human body. They account for a sixth of our body weight. Fats are organic compounds that are composed of carbon, hydrogen and oxygen. These are also major sources of energy. Fats belong to a group of substances called lipids, are the combinations of saturated and unsaturated fatty acids.

Classification of fats

Fats are classified as:

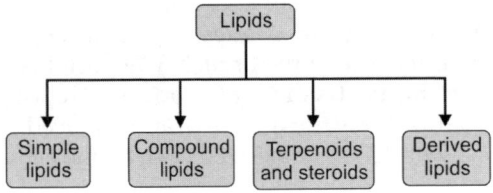

- *Simple Lipids*
    1. **Triglycerides, neutral fats:** Esters of three molecules of fatty acids combining glycerol to form triglycerides. These are found in adipose tissue, butterfat, lard, suet, fish oils, olive oil, corn oil, *etc.*
    2. **Waxes:** Waxes are composed of esters of fatty acids with alcohol other than glycerol. Waxes are found in beeswax, head oil of sperm whale, cerumen, carnauba oil and lanolin.

- *Compound Lipids*
    1. **Phospholipids (phosphatides):** Phospholipids are composed of glycerol, fatty acids and phosphoric acid bound in ester linkage to a nitrogenous base.

Phospholipids are found chiefly in animal tissues.

2. **Lecithin:** Lecithin is important for fat metabolism and transportation. Lecithins are found in brain, egg yolk and organ meats. These are used as emulsifying agents in the food industry.

3. **Cephalin:** Cephalin occurs predominantly in nervous tissue.

4. **Plasmalogen:** Found in brain, heart, and muscle.

5. **Lipositol:** Found in brain, heart, kidneys and plant tissues together with phytic acid.

6. **Sphingomyelin:** Found in nervous tissue, brain and red blood cells. Sphingosine-containing phosphatide, yields fatty acids, choline, sphingosine and phosphoric acid. These are important sources of phosphoric acid in body tissue.

7. **Glycolipids:**
    a. *Cerebroside*: The hydrolysis of fatty acids yield cerebroside. Cerebrosides are present in myline sheaths of nerves, brain and other tissues.
    b. *Ganglioside*: Gangliosides are found in brain, nerve tissue and other tissues, such as spleen. Gangliosides provide the carbohydrates determinants of the human blood groups A, B and O.
    c. *Sulfolipid*: Sulfur-containing glycolipid; sulfate present in ester linkage to galactose. Sulfolipids are present in white matter of brain, liver and testicle. These are also present in plant chloroplast.

d. *Proteolipids*: Proteolipids are complexes of protein and lipids. These are present in brain and nerve tissue.

- *Steroids*

  Sterols:

  a. *Cholesterol*: A consituent of bile acids and a precursor of vitamin D. Cholesterol is found in egg yolk, dairy products and animal tissues.

  b. *Ergosterol*: Converted to vitamin D_2 on irradiation. Ergosterol is found in plant tissues, yeast and fungi.

  c. *7-dehydrocholesterol*: Converted to D_3 on irradiation. This is found in animal tissues and underneath skin.

- *Derived lipids*

  Fatty acids: Fatty acids contain a number of carbon atoms and are straight chain derivatives.

  Fatty acids are classified into two types:

  i. **Saturated fats:** These are the biggest dietary cause of high LDL levels ("bad cholesterol"). Saturated fats are found in animal products such as butter, cheese, whole milk, ice cream, cream and fatty meats. These are also found in some vegetable oils— coconut, palm and palm kernel oils.

  ii. **Unsaturated fats:** Unsaturated fats have a single bond between its carbon atoms. These are considered as healthy fats as these fats help in lowering blood cholesterol, if used in place of saturated fats. Most (but not all) liquid vegetable oils are unsaturated. The oils not containing unsaturated fats include coconut, palm and palm kernel oils. There are two types of unsaturated fats:

     - **Monounsaturated fats:** They have only one double bond in the molecules. Examples include olive and canola oils.

     - **Polyunsaturated fats:** They have two or more double bonds in the molecules. Examples include fish, safflower, sunflower, corn and soybean oils.

Functions of Fats

Fats provide energy: Fats also provide energy. 1 gm of fats yields 9 gm of energy for the body compared with four calories per gram of carbohydrates and proteins. Fats are stored within most cells but a large amount of fat is stored in a large number of specialized fat cells called adipocytes within adipose tissue whose function is to store fat thus provides energy when needed.

Fats build healthy cells: Fats are vital part of the membrane that surrounds each cell of the body. Without a healthy cell membrane, the rest of the cell couldn't function.

Fats build brains: Fat provides the structural components not only of cell membranes in the brain, but also of myelin, the fatty insulating sheath that surrounds each nerve fibre, enabling it to carry messages faster.

Fats are the sources of vitamins: Fats contain vitamins A, D, E and K which are absorbed by the intestine and play vital role in various functions in the body.

Fats help in synthesis of hormones: Fats are structural components of some of the most important substances in the body, including prostaglandins, hormone-like substances that regulate many of the body's functions. Fats regulate the production of sex hormones, which are involved in promoting conception, inducing labor, effecting spontaneous abortion and regulating blood pressure.

Fat makes skin healthier: The deficiency of fats makes skin to look dry and flaky. In addition to give the skin a healthy appearance, the layer of fat, just beneath the skin (called subcutaneous fat) acts as the body's own insulation to help in regulating body temperature.

Fat forms a protective cushion for your organs: Fats also help the organ from shocks as many of the vital organs, especially the kidneys, heart and intestines are cushioned by fat that helps to protect them from injury and hold them in place.

Fats are essential for brain: Fat provides the structural components not only of cell membranes in the brain, but also of myelin, the fatty insulating sheath that surrounds each nerve fibre, enabling it to carry messages faster.

Sources of fats: Whole milk, meat, butter, oils, ghee, eggs, corn, olives, meat, nuts, peanuts, avocado, shredded coconut, cream, cheese, all are sources of fats.

VITAMINS

Vitamins are essential nutrients for human beings. Vitamins are used by the body to stay healthy and support its many functions. Vitamins do not provide energy (calories) directly, but they do help to regulate energy-producing processes. With the exception of vitamins D and K, vitamins cannot be synthesized by the human body and must be obtained from the diet. Vitamins have to come from food because they are not manufactured or formed by the body.

Types of Vitamins

Water-soluble Vitamins

Water-soluble vitamins are easily absorbed by the body. These vitamins are easily destroyed or washed out during food storage and preparation. They are eliminated in urine so, body needs a continuous supply of them in diets.

Vitamin B, which includes B_1, B_2, B_3, B_5, B_6, B_7, B_9 and B_{12} and vitamin C (ascorbic acid) are water-soluble vitamins. The chemical names of B vitamins are B_1 (thiamine), B_2 is riboflavin, B_3 is niacin, B_5 is pantothenic acid, B_6 is pyridoxine, B_7 is biotin, B_9 is folic acid, and B_{12} is cyanocobalamin which are widely distributed in foods.

Fat-soluble Vitamins

The vitamins A, D, E and K are fat soluble vitamins. As the name indicates these are soluble in fat and are absorbed by the body from the intestinal tract. The human body has to use bile acids to absorb fat-soluble vitamins. Once these vitamins are absorbed, the body stores them in body fat. When you need them,

your body takes them out of storage to be used. Eating fats or oils that are not digested can cause lack of fat-soluble vitamins.

Functions of water-soluble vitamins

Vitamin B_1 (thiamine)

Thiamine is one of the important B-vitamins which are involved in various functions of the body. It enhances blood circulation and helps in blood formation and the metabolism of carbohydrates. It is also required for the health of the nervous system and is used in the biosynthesis of a number of cell constituents, including the neurotransmitter acetylcholine and gamma-amino butyric acid (GABA). It is also involved in the manufacture of hydrochloric acid, and therefore plays an important role in digestion.

It is also important for the development of brain and helps in removing depression and enhances memory and learning. In children it is required for growth and has shown some indication to assist in arthritis, cataracts as well as infertility.

Chemical structure of B_1 (thiamine)

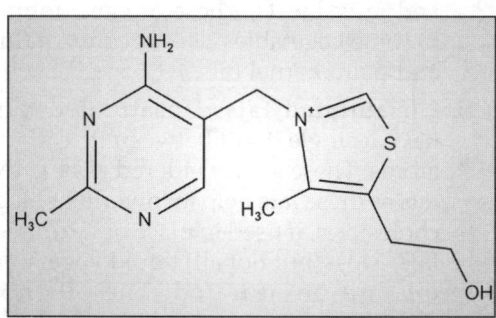

Deficiency disorders: The lack of thiamine in the diet causes Beriberi, a disease of nervous system. Besides this, the deficiency of this vitamin may also cause tiredness and fatigue, muscle weakness, nerve damage, confusion and enlarged heart.

Food sources of vitamin B_1: Asparagus, wheat germ, brown rice, rice bran, oatmeal, legumes, peanuts, sunflower seeds and dried soybeans. Nuts such as pistachio nuts, raw peanuts, dried pecans, and raisins and vegetables such as peas, millet, cabbage, broccoli, are excellent sources. Meat products like poultry, pork, liver, kidney and fish are excellent sources of vitamin B_1.

Vitamin B_2 (riboflavin)

Vitamin B_2 is important for conversion of riboflavin to flavin mononucleotide (FMN) and further to the predominant flavin adenine dinucleotide (FAD) occurs before these flavins form complexes with numerous flavoprotein dehydrogenases and oxidases. These flavocoenzymes (FMN and FASD) participate in oxidation–reduction reactions in metabolic pathways and in energy production via the respiratory chain. It is important for body growth and red blood cell production and helps in releasing energy from carbohydrates. It prevents constipation, promotes a healthy skin, nails and hair, and strengthens the mucous lining of the mouth, lips and tongue. Riboflavin aids digestion and helps in the functioning of the nervous system.

Chemical structure of vitamin B_2

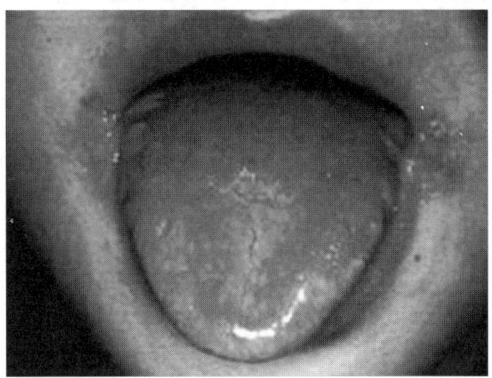

Deficiency disorders: The deficiency of this vitamin leads to angular stomatitis (the lesions at the angles of the mouth), cheilosis (dry chapped appearance of the lips as shown in figure), behavioural abnormalities occur in riboflavin deficient childreny.

Food sources: The foods such as dairy products, eggs, green leafy vegetables, lean meats, legumes, milk and nuts provide riboflavin in the diet. Breads and cereals are often fortified with riboflavin. Fortified means the vitamin has been added to the food.

Vitamin B_3 (niacin)

Niacin is important for heart and prevents arteriosclerosis. Niacin helps in lowering blood levels of "bad" LDL (Low Density Lipoprotein) cholesterol and preventing the accumulation of arterial plaque. Niacin is also important for digestive system, nervous system and brain, to function well. Niacin is also involved in the formation of new DNA, and is also involved in controlling the blood sugar levels as it helps the body to use insulin efficiently. Niacin also has a number of therapeutic uses. It also helps to treat arthritis, diabetes and acne, as well as mental disorders like dementia, schizophrenia and psychosis.

Chemical structure of B_3 (niacin)

Deficiency disorders: The deficiency may lead to skin disorders, fatigue, depression and diarrhea, glossitis and dermatitis.

Food sources of vitamin B$_3$: The best food sources of vitamin B$_3$ are found in beets, beef liver, beef kidney, fish, salmon, swordfish, tuna, sunflower seeds and peanuts. Bread and cereals are usually fortified with niacin. In addition, foods that contain tryptophan and an amino acid, the body converts it into niacin include poultry, red meat, eggs and dairy products.

Vitamin B$_5$ (pantothenic acid)

Pantothenic acid acts as coenzyme A and is also known as "antistress" vitamin. It is closely involved in adrenal cortex function. It supports the adrenal glands to increase production of cortisone and other adrenal hormones to help counteract stress and enhance metabolism. Through this mechanism, pantothenic acid is also thought to help prevent of aging and wrinkles. It is generally important to healthy skin and nerves. Through its adrenal support, vitamin B$_5$ may reduce potentially toxic effects of antibiotics and radiation.

As the coenzyme, pantothenic acid is important in cellular metabolism of carbohydrates and fats to release energy. As coenzyme A, it supports the synthesis of acetylcholine, a very important neurotransmitter agent that works throughout the body in a variety of neuromuscular reactions. Coenzyme A is vital in the synthesis of fatty acids, cholesterol, steroids, sphingosines and phospholipids. It also helps to synthesize porphyrin, which is connected to hemoglobin.

Chemical structure of B$_5$ (pantothenic acid)

Deficiency disorders: A deficiency causes tiredness and a loss of feeling in the toes. The visible signs of deficiency include nausea, vomiting, tremor of the outstretched hands and irritability.

Food sources: Beef liver, milk, eggs, rice, mushrooms and potatoes are good sources of pantothenic acid.

Vitamin B$_6$ (pyridoxine)

Pyridoxine assists in the balancing of sodium and potassium as well as promoting red blood cell production. It is linked to cardiovascular health by decreasing the formation of homocysteine. Pyridoxine may help to balance hormonal changes in women and aids the immune system.

It is required for the production of the monoamine neurotransmitters serotonin, dopamine, norepinephrine and epinephrine, as it is the precursor to pyridoxal phosphate— cofactor for the enzyme aromatic amino acid decarboxylase. This enzyme is responsible for converting the precursors 5-hydroxy-tryptophan (5-HTP) into serotonin and levodopa (L-DOPA) into dopamine, nora-drenaline and adrenaline.

Chemical structure of B$_6$ (pyridoxine)

Deficiency disorder: Lack of pyridoxine may cause anemia, nerve damage, seizures, skin problems and sores in the mouth.

Food sources: Spinach, cereals, turkey, brown rice, sweet potatoes, turnip and liver are the good sources of pyridoxine.

Vitamin B$_7$ (biotin)

Vitamin B$_7$ also called vitamin H, helps the nervous system functions properly, as well as helps to promote healthy skin and hair. Biotin may help to fight for alopecia, a form of hair loss. This vitamin is also necessary for healthy embryonic growth during pregnancy. The vitamin could help in strengthening the brittleness of nails.

Deficiency disorder: The deficiency of biotin may cause hair loss or brittle hair, skin rashes and fungal infection. This could lead to depression and muscular pain.

Food sources: Onions, cucumbers, cauliflower, strawberries, raspberries, goat's milk, cow's milk, carrots, almonds, walnuts, eggs, liver, soyabean and whole wheat bread are the good sources of biotin.

Vitamin B$_9$ (folic acid)

Folic acid is crucial for proper brain function and plays an important role in mental and emotional health. It aids in the production of DNA and RNA, the body's genetic material, and is especially important when cells and tissues are growing rapidly, such as in infancy, adolescence and pregnancy. Folic acid also works closely with vitamin B$_{12}$ to help in making red blood cells and help iron to work properly in the body.

Chemical structure of B$_9$ (Folic acid)

Deficiency disorder: The deficiency of folic acid leads to anemia, incorrect absorption of essential nutrients and neural tube defects (abnormal development of the neural tube) in babies, spina bifida, poor growth, tongue inflammation, gingivitis, loss of appetite, shortness of breath, diarrhea, irritability, forgetfulness and mental sluggishness.

Food sources: Cereals, beans and legumes, green leafy vegetables, kidney beans, sunflower seeds, peanuts, asparagus, corn, cauliflower, potatoes, beets, orange juice, tomato juice, cantaloupe, avocados and soya milk contains this essential vitamin B$_9$.

Vitamin B$_{12}$ (cyanocobalamin)

Cyanocobalamin is essential for the production and regeneration of red blood cells. Vitamin B$_{12}$ is necessary for proper utilization of fats, carbohydrates and proteins for body building.

It is also needed for the proper functioning of the central nervous system. It improves concentration, memory and balance, and relieves irritability. It promotes growth and increases appetite in children. This vitamin is also involved in metabolism of folic acid.

Chemical structure of B$_{12}$ (cyanocobalamin)

Deficiency disorders: Tiredness and fatigue, tingling and numbness in the hands and feet, loss of memory, pernicious anemia and confusion.

Food sources: Milk, cheese, fish, shellfish, organ meats, particularly liver and kidney, eggs, beef and pork contain cyanocobalamin.

Vitamin C (ascorbic acid)

The most prominent role of vitamin C is its immune-stimulating effect, which is important for defense against infections such as common colds. It also acts as an inhibitor of histamine, a compound that is released during allergic reactions. As a powerful antioxidant, it can neutralize harmful free radicals and it aids in neutralizing pollutants and toxins. Thus it is able to prevent the formation of potentially carcinogenic nitrosamines in the stomach (due to consumption of nitrite-containing foods, such as smoked meat).

Importantly, vitamin C is also able to regenerate other antioxidants such as vitamin E. Vitamin C is required for the synthesis of collagen, the intercellular "cement" substance which gives structure to muscles, vascular tissues, bones, tendons and ligaments. Vitamin C in combination with zinc helps in the healing of wounds.

In addition, vitamin C contributes to the health of teeth and gums, preventing hemorrhaging and bleeding. It also improves the absorption of iron from the diet. Vitamin C is also needed for the metabolism of bile acids which may have implications for blood cholesterol levels and gallstones. Moreover, vitamin C plays an important role in the synthesis of several important peptide hormones, neurotransmitters and carnitine.

Deficiency disorders: The deficiency of the vitamin may cause infections, slower healing of wounds, dental and gum problems, fatigue, loss of appetite, dry skin, painful joints, anemia and a slower metabolism.

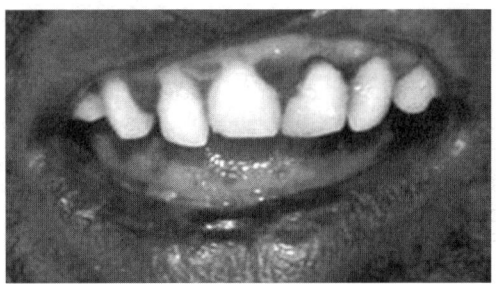

Scurvy caused due to deficiency of vitamin C

Chemical structure of vitamin C (ascorbic acid)

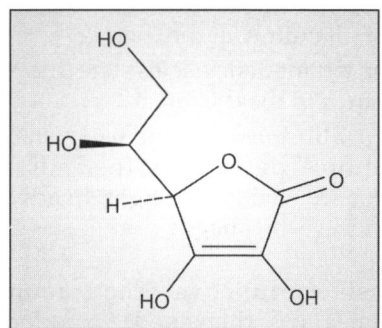

Food sources: Vitamin C is present in broccoli, sprouts, cauliflower, lemon juice, strawberries, mustard greens, papaya, amla, cabbage, turnip greens, oranges, cantaloupe, summer squash, grapefruit, pineapple, tomatoes, collard greens, raspberries, spinach, green beans, fennel, asparagus and watermelon.

Functions of fat-soluble vitamins

Vitamin A (retinol)

Vitamin A also helps to keep skin and mucous membranes that line the nose, sinuses, and mouth healthy. It plays a role in immune system function, growth, bone formation, reproduction, and wound healing.

Vitamin A comes from two sources. One group comes from animal sources and is called retinoids, which includes retinol. The other group comes from plants and is called carotenoids, which includes beta-carotene. The body converts beta-carotene to vitamin A.

Chemical structure of vitamin A

Deficiency disorders: Poor night vision, eye problems, weakened immune system and more prone to infection occurs due to deficiency of vitamin A in the diet.

The important deficiencies state due to lack of vitamin A in the diet are:

i. **Night blindness:** In the early stages of vitamin A deficiency, the individual cannot see well in dim light. In advanced deficiency, the subject cannot see objects in dim light.

ii. **Xerosis conjunctiva:** The conjunctiva becomes dry, thickened, wrinkled and pigmented. The pigmentation gives conjunctiva a smoky appearance.

iii. **Xerosis cornea:** When dryness spreads to cornea, it takes on a hazy, lusterless appearance.

iv. **Bitot's spots:** Greyish glistening white plaques formed of desquamated thickened conjuctival epithelium, usually triangular in shape and firmly adhering to the conjuctiva.

v. **Keratomalacia:** When xerosis of the conjuctiva and cornea is not treated, it may develop into a condition known as keratomalacia.

vi. **Follicular hyperkeratosis:** The skin becomes rough and dry.

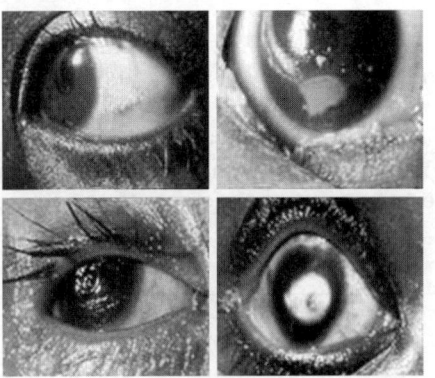

Under the national prophylaxis programme against nutritional blindness 2,00,000 IU of vitamin A in oil is administered on every six months to preschool children to eliminate vitamin A deficiency.

Food sources: Eggs are good sources of vitamin A and other nutrients and advocated as a measure to prevent vitamin A deficiency. Green leafy vegetables and yellow orange fruits and vegetables like mango, papaya and carrots are rich sources of vitamin A.

Vitamin D (calciferol)

Vitamin D is now considered more a prohormone than a vitamin. It can be synthesized in the body in adequate amounts by simple exposure to sunlight.

The main function of vitamin D is to keep normal calcium and phosphorus levels in the body which helps to maintain and build strong bones, teeth and nails. Also it supports cell functions and other neuromuscular functions in the body. By controlling the supply of calcium between the bones and the blood, it supports bone mineralization (hardening of bones) and bone remodeling by osteoblasts and osteoclasts. Vitamin D also plays a substantial role in preventing rickets in children, and osteoporosis or osteomalacia in adults. Being a powerful antioxidant and anti-carcinogen, it helps in combating depression, prostate cancer, breast cancer, high blood pressure, cardiovascular diseases, phagocytosis activity and boosts anti-tumor activity. Vitamin D also helps treating conditions like diabetes and obesity, and prevents the onset of multiple sclerosis. Hence, we can say vitamin D helps in maintaining a healthy immune system and is important for body's overall growth and development.

Chemical structure of vitamin D

CH₃ ... H₃C ... CH₃ ... H₃C ... CH₃ ... H ... H ... Calciferol (D2) ... CH₂ ... HO

Deficiency disorders: Softening and weakening of the bones that are rickets in children and osteomalacia in adults, insomnia, nervousness and muscle weakness.

Rickets: Rickets is most severe in the children between 1 and 3 years, which leads to softening and weakening of the bones.

Signs of Rickets

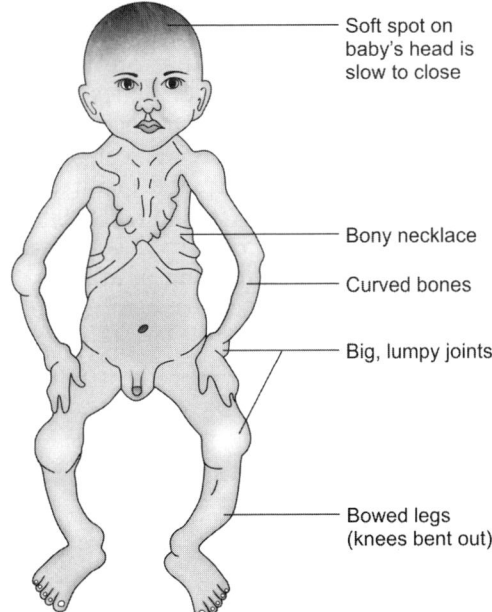

Soft spot on baby's head is slow to close

Bony necklace

Curved bones

Big, lumpy joints

Bowed legs (knees bent out)

Osteomalacia: It may be called adult rickets. It occurs generally in pregnant women. The changes in bone are similar to rickets. Skeletal pain is usually present and persistent and ranges from a dull ache to severe pain. Muscular weakness is often present and the patient may find difficulty in climbing stairs or getting out of a chair.

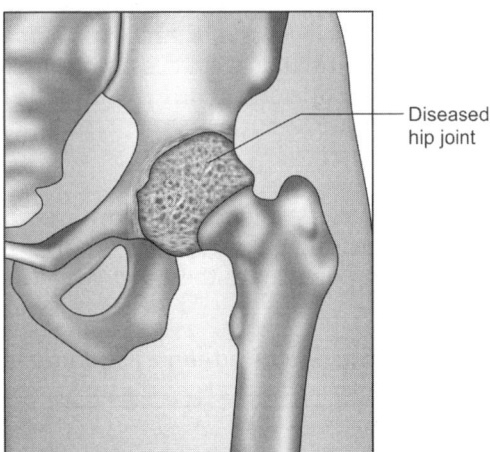

Diseased hip joint

Food sources: Marine fishes are known to be good sources of vitamin D. Egg yolk, butter and milk have some vitamin D and can be considered as poor sources. Recent work indicated that the fresh water fishes have moderate amounts of vitamin D_3 in liver.

Vitamin E (tocopherol)

Vitamin E is an important antioxidant that protects the cells and tissues from harmful substances and free radicals. Vitamin E is believed to help delay or prevent heart disease by protecting the walls of the arteries. It prevents bad cholesterol (LDL) from being oxidized, preventing clogged arteries and some types of cancer. Vitamin E can also prevent platelets from clumping together and forming blood clots. This can help to prevent a stroke or heart attack. Vitamin E can also help to fight cancer. It protects the cell's DNA from damage that can cause the cells to turn cancerous. It reduces the rate of growth for tumors, at the same time enhancing the immune system to fight cancer. Vitamin E also enhances the action of insulin. This improves blood glucose function in diabetes. It also plays a pivotal role in the proper function of the brain. It protects the myelin sheaths that surround neurons in the brain. This can help to prevent degeneration during the normal aging process. It may also help to prevent Alzheimer's disease. Vitamin E can also be used to reduce or clear scars on the skin, including acne scars.

Chemical structure of vitamin E (tocopherol)

Deficiency disorders: Deficiency may lead to nerve damage, cystic fibrosis, isolated vitamin E deficiency syndrome, dry hair or loss of hair, muscular weakness, slow tissue healing, reproduction failure and liver necrosis.

Food sources: Almonds, sunflower seeds, wheat germ oil, peanut butter, corn oil, spinach and papaya are the good sources of vitamin E.

Vitamin K (phylloquinone)

Vitamin K is important for blood clotting, if major injury happens. Vitamin K plays a necessary role in synthesis of several proteins that mediate both coagulation and anti-coagulation. Vitamin K deficiency leads to bleeding excessively. It also helps to maintain strong bones and could prevent osteoporosis. It improves bone density and facilitates the absorption of calcium. Vitamin K also helps in reducing the risk of coronary heart diseases by preventing the hardening of arteries.

Chemical structure of vitamin K (phylloquinone)

Deficiency disorders: The deficiency of vitamin K leads to nose bleeding, gum bleeding, heavy menstrual bleeding in women, hematuria, intercranial hemorrhage and gastrointestinal bleeding.

As vitamin K is essential to the process of bone formation and repair, bone density and the absorption of calcium by the bone, vitamin K deficiency can cause weak bones and osteoporosis. Vitamin K is emerging as a potential protector against osteoporosis, atherosclerosis, insulin sensitivity and cancer.

Food sources: The concentration of vitamin K in foods is highest in dark green leafy vegetables but is also found in fruits, tubers, seeds and dairy and meat products.

MINERALS

Minerals are natural compounds which are needed by the body in small amounts to help it function properly and stay strong. Minerals are important for maintaining the normal body functions and regulatory processes.

The important minerals that are essential to human health are: Calcium, phosphorus, magnesium, sodium, potassium, chloride, sulfur, iron, manganese, copper, iodine, zinc, fluoride and selenium. These 14 essential minerals are essential for the growth and production of bones, teeth, hair, blood, nerves, skin, vitamins, enzymes and hormones and the healthy functioning of nerve transmission, blood circulation, fluid regulation, cellular integrity, energy production and muscle contraction.

Types of minerals: There are two types of minerals:

1. Macro minerals
2. Micro minerals
1. **Macro minerals:** Macro minerals are dietary minerals that are needed by the human body in high quantities. The macro mineral group includes calcium, phosphorus, magnesium, sodium and potassium.
2. **Micro or trace minerals:** Micro minerals, also known as trace elements that are needed in very little amount. Trace minerals include iron, manganese, copper, iodine, zinc, fluoride and selenium.

Macro Minerals

Calcium

Calcium is the most abundant mineral in the human body and has several important functions. Calcium is an important mineral which helps in building strong bones, and is a primary structural constituent of the skeleton, but it is also widely distributed in soft tissues where it is involved in neuro-muscular, enzymatic, hormonal and other metabolic activities.

Calcium absorption is dependent upon the calcium needs of the body, the foods eaten, and the amount of calcium in the foods eaten. Vitamin D from diet or exposure to the ultraviolet light of the sun increases calcium absorption. Calcium absorption tends to decrease with increased age for both men and women. More than 99% of total body calcium is stored in the bones and teeth where it functions to support their structure. The remaining 1% is found throughout the body in blood, muscle and the fluid between cells. Because of its biological importance, calcium levels are carefully controlled in various compartments of the body. The three major regulators of blood calcium are parathyroid hormone (PTH), vitamin D and calcitonin.

Functionality of calcium:

- Calcium is important for building of strong bones and healthy teeth.
- Calcium is also used in muscle contraction, blood clotting, and maintenance of cell membranes.
- About 1% of the total body pool of calcium is utilized to support nerve transmission, muscle contraction (including normal heart rhythm), blood clotting, and regulation of enzyme and hormone activities.
- Membrane calcium transport systems are involved in regulation of cellular osmolarity and peripheral vascular resistance.
- Calcium is important for production of milk during pregnancy and nursing period.

Deficiency diseases of calcium: Arthritis, high blood pressure and osteoporosis.

Table 5.2: The differential diagnosis of osteomalacia and osteoporosis

Features	Osteomalacia	Osteoporosis
General		
Type	It is a deficiency disease.	It is not a primary deficiency.
Age at which it occurs	It occurs in the reproductive stage due to repeated pregnancies.	It occurs in the post menopausal stage.
Composition of bone	Composition of bone changes. Amount of calcium and phosphorous is low and bone become translucent	Composition of bone remains the same. Decrease in quantity of the bone
Deficiency	Less accretion of calcium and phosphorous in the bone due to the deficiency of vitamin D	Resorption of the bone is more due to the deficiency of estrogen.
Sex	It occurs mostly in women.	It occurs mostly in women but men can also get it.
Clinical features		
Skeletal pain	A major complaint usually persistent	Episodic and usually associated with a fracture
Muscle weakness	Usually present and producing disability and when severe, a characteristic gait	Absent
Fractures	Relatively uncommon; healing delayed	The usual presenting feature; heals normally
Skeletal deformity	Common, especially kyphos	Only occurs where there is a fracture
Radiographic features		
Loss of density of bone	Widespread	Irregular and often most marked in the spine
Looser's zones (Rarefaction of bone and translucent bands)	Diagnostic	Absent
Biopsy		
Histological changes	Excess osteoic' tissue with bone present in normal quantity	Bone reduced in quantity but fully mineralized
Biochemical changes		
Plasma Ca and P	Often low	Normal
Plasma alkaline phosphatase	Often high	Normal
Urinary calcium Response to treatment	Often low	Normal or high
Vitamin D	Dramatic	None

Source: (Modified) Passmore R and Eastwood MA, 1990. Davidson and Passmore, Human nutrition and dietetics, Modified ELBS, Churchill Livingstone.

Rich sources of calcium:

- Dairy products, such as milk, cheese and yoghurt
- Canned salmon and sardines with bones
- Leafy green vegetables, such as broccoli, spinach
- Calcium-fortified foods — from orange juice to cereals and crackers
- Ice cream, oysters

Recommended daily intake: The recommended daily intakes (RDI) for calcium is shown in the table given below:

Calcium requirements	
Life stage	Calcium mg/day
Infants	
0–6 months	210
7–12 months	270
Children	
1–3 years	500
4–8 years	800
Males	
9–13 years	1300
14–18 years	1300
19–30 years	1000
31–50 years	1000
51–70 years	1200
>70 years	1200
Females	
9–13 years	1300
14–18 years	1300
19–30 years	1000
31–50 years	1000
51–70 years	1200
>70 years	1200
Pregnancy	
< 18 years	1300
19–30 years	1000
31–50 years	1000
Lactation	
< 18 years	1300
19–30 years	1000
31–50 years	1000

Phosphorus

Phosphorus is the second most abundant mineral in the body and 85% of it is found in the bones. The rest of the body's phosphorus is found in the blood. It is found in the body usually at a ratio of 1:2 to calcium. It is a nonmetallic element that is found in the blood, muscles, nerves, bones and teeth and is a component of adenosine tri-phosphate

Functionality of phosphorus: The main functions of phosphorus are as follows:

- Phosphorus helps to maintain normal acid-base balance (pH) in its role as one of the body's most important buffers.
- It plays an important role in the growth, maintenance, and repair of cells.
- It maintains the pH level (acidity-alkalinity) of the blood.
- It helps in reducing the pain of arthritis.
- It is essential for speedy recovery of burn victims.
- Helps in cancer prevention.
- It is essential for building of strong bones and skeletal structure.
- It maintains heart regularity.

Deficiency diseases: Rickets, osteoporosis, stiff joints and pain in the bones. The deficiency can also cause anxiety, irritability, sensitive skin, stress, tiredness and weak teeth, *etc.*

Rich sources: Milk, yoghurt, cottage cheese, American cheese, pork, hamburger, tuna, lobster, chicken, sunflower seeds, peanuts, pine nuts, peanut butter, bran flakes, shredded wheat, whole wheat bread, noodles, rice, white bread, potatoes, corn, peas, french fries, broccoli, milk chocolate and soda beverages (due to the phosphoric acid added as a preservative).

Recommended daily intake:

- Men and women: 1000 mg
  Phosphorus is best taken as part of a multivitamin and mineral supplement.

Magnesium

Magnesium is one of the families of major minerals although, it is not as well known as some of the other minerals in the same group. Even though it is not as prominent, the magnesium mineral plays an essential role in about three hundred biochemical processes that take place inside the body.

Functionality of magnesium:

- It is essential to maintain both the acid-alkaline balance in the body and healthy functioning of nerves and muscles.
- Potassium helps in lowering the high blood pressure.
- Promotes healthy cardiovascular system to prevent heart disease and arrhythmia.
- Calcium deposits, kidney stones, and gall-stones.
- Relief from indigestion
  i. Inhibits blood clots and widens arteries
  ii. Diabetes prevention
  iii. Relaxes muscles and reduces severity of asthma by widening the airways.

Deficiency diseases: Heart disease, diabetes and osteoporosis.

Overdose disease: Kidney failure

Deficiency symptoms:

- Nausea
- Vomiting
- Loss of appetite
- Fatigue and a feeling of weakness

Rich sources: Dark green vegetables such as spinach, kale, broccoli and avocado are excellent magnesium sources. Other magnesium sources include whole grains, legumes, black beans, brown rice, lentils, almonds, cashews, peanuts and peanut butter, bananas, soyabeans, wheat bran and bran flakes, lean meats, dry figs, halibut, crab and sardines.

Best suitable composition: It is best taken with calcium, iron, B group vitamins as well as vitamin E.

Recommended daily intake:

- Children: 80–240 mg
- Men: 350 mg
- Women: 300 mg
- Pregnancy: 350–400 mg
- Breastfeeding: 310–360 mg

Potassium

Potassium is the third most abundant mineral in the body and is considered as electrolyte.

Potassium keeps your muscles and nervous system working properly.

Functionality of potassium:

- Potassium is needed for growth, building muscles, transmission of nerve impulses, heart activity, *etc.*
- It assists in muscle contractions and in maintaining appropriate levels of fluid and the electrolyte balance in the body cells.
- Potassium also plays an important role in the conduction of nerve impulses and enables the body to convert glucose into energy, which is then stored in reserve by the muscles and liver.
- Potassium is essential for maintaining fluid balance in the body.

Deficiency diseases: Fatigue, cramping legs, muscle weakness, slow reflexes, acne, dry skin, mood changes and irregular heartbeat.

Overdose disease: Kidney failure

Deficiency symptoms:

- Weakness
- Scarring of heart muscle, irregular heartbeat or heart failure
- Hypertrophy of kidneys
- Paralysis of muscle
- Retarded bone growth

Rich sources: Bananas, broccoli, tomatoes, potatoes with skins, kiwi, leafy green vegetables, broccoli citrus fruits, oranges, dried fruits, dates, apricots, avocado, beans, peas, lentils, and peanuts are rich sources of potassium.

Best suitable composition: A person should take as much potassium as sodium twice, and is best taken with vitamin B_6.

Recommended daily intake:

- Men and women: 3500 mg

Sodium

Sodium is another important mineral which is involved in various functions of the body.

Functionality of sodium:

- Sodium is important for the manufacture of hydrochloric acid in the stomach, which protects the body from any infections that may be present in food.

- It is required for maintaining blood pressure.
- The important function of sodium is to regulate fluids and acid-base balance in the body.
- Sodium is required for nerve transmission and muscle contraction.
- Sodium is important for treatment of diarrhea, leg cramps, dehydration and fever.

Deficiency diseases: Diarrhea and vomiting

Overdose disease: High blood pressure and hypertension

Deficiency symptoms:

Sodium is an important part of water, hence deficiency of water in the body may cause:

- Muscle cramps and weakness
- Dizziness
- Inability to concentrate
- Memory impairment and nausea

Rich sources: Sodium is found in table salt, ajinomoto, sauces, *etc.*

Recommended daily intake:

- Men and women: 2400 mg

Micro Minerals

Iron

Iron is the most important component of blood which is regarded as the oxygen-carrying component of the blood. It is stored as ferritin which is a soluble iron-storage compound. The most important function of iron is the formation of hemoglobin, which is the part of red blood cells that carries oxygen throughout the body. Iron is also found in myoglobin, which distributes oxygen to the muscle, skeletal, and heart muscles. Iron is also important for the proper functioning of the immune system and the production of energy.

Functionality of iron: The important functions of iron are as follows:

- Iron is needed for the transportation of oxygen from lungs to the body.

- It is necessary for the formation of hemo-globin.
- It is important for proper brain development.
- Iron helps in the regulation of body temperature.
- Iron is required for the binding of oxygen to the blood cells.

Deficiency diseases: Anemia

Overdose disease: Cancer, liver and heart damage, diabetes and skin changes

Deficiency symptoms:

- Lethargy, poor concentration
- Pale skin and shortness of breath
- Poor stamina
- Intestinal bleeding
- Excessive menstrual bleeding
- Nervousness
- Heart palpitations

Rich sources: Iron is found in meat, fish, beans, spinach, molasses, kelp, brewer's yeast, broccoli and seeds. Many common herbs, such as thyme, turmeric and cumin seeds are high in iron.

Recommended daily intake:

- Men: 10 mg
- Women: 18 mg

Zinc

Zinc is an essential trace element which is important for the normal growth, development, reproduction and immunity. It is required for the synthesis of protein and collagen — which is important for wound healing and a healthy skin. Zinc is also found to be important for maintaining a healthy appetite and for good vision.

Functionality of zinc:

- It helps in enhancing the immunity, thus prevents infections.
- It also helps in cell growth and healing of wounds.
- It helps in formation of proteins and genetic material.
- Zinc is involved in transportation of cholesterol and maintaining the stability of lipids within the cell membrane.

- Fighting skin problems such as acne, boils and sore throats
- Zinc is important for sexual development.
- It is involved in synthesis of protein.

Deficiency diseases: The deficiency of zinc in the body leads to:

1. Allergies
2. Night blindness
3. Loss of smell
4. Falling hair
5. White spots under fingernails
6. Skin problems
7. Sleep disturbances

Overdose disease: Nausea, diarrhea, dizziness, drowsiness and hallucinations may occur due to over intake of zinc in the diet.

Deficiency symptoms:
- Hair loss
- Diarrhoea
- Fatigue
- Delayed wound healing
- Decreased mental development in infants

Rich sources: The good sources of zinc are beef, black beans, chicken heart, egg yolk, fish, lamb, maple syrup, milk, nuts, pork, sesame seeds, soyabeans, sunflower seeds, turkey, wheat germ, whole grain products and yeast.

Recommended daily intake:
- Men: 15 mg
- Women: 12 mg

Manganese

Manganese is found mostly in bones, liver, kidneys and pancreas. Manganese helps the body form connective tissue, bones, blood clotting factors and sex hormones. It also plays a role in fat and carbohydrate metabolism, calcium absorption, and blood sugar regulation. Manganese is also necessary for normal brain and nerve function and also helps in preventing free radical formation.

Deficiency diseases: Problems with the disks between the vertebrae, birth defects, and problems with blood glucose levels and reduced fertility.

Serious deficiency in children can result in paralysis, deafness and blindness.

Overdose disease: Manganese madness

Deficiency symptoms: Symptoms include:
- Seizures
- Epilepsy
- Poor muscle coordination
- Facial twitching
- Bone deformities
- Weakness
- Deficiencies in children may lead to stunted growth and development.

Rich sources: Nuts, green leafy vegetables, peas, beets, egg yolks, whole grain cereals, organ meats, bran, fruits and black tea.

Recommended daily intake:
- Men and women: 2.5–5 mg

Copper

Copper is the third most abundant trace mineral in the body. It is also a part of many enzyme systems. Copper is also important for the formation and regulation of hormones such as melatonin and for the production of a wide range of neurotransmitters and other neuroactive compounds, including the catecholamines and encephalins.

Functionality of copper:
- Copper is important for the formation of collagen.
- Copper is important component of cytochrome oxidase-controls intracellular energy production.
- It helps in controlling various hormone levels in the body.
- Prevents free radical formation.
- Copper is important for fatty acid metabolism.
- It helps in maintaining the normal haemoglobin level in the body.

Deficiency diseases: The deficiency of copper leads to Menkes syndrome, Wilson's disease, kwashiorkor and neutropenia.

Overdose disease: Diarrhea, vomiting, liver damage as well as discoloration of the skin and hair.

Deficiency symptoms:
- Changes in hair colour and texture
- Hair loss

- Disturbances to the nervous system
- Bone diseases
- Immune system dysfunction
- Vascular disease (hemorrhage in severe cases)
- Brittle bones (in children)
- Oedema (swelling)
- High cholesterol levels
- Poorly pigmented skin
- Anemia

Rich sources: Good sources include cocoa, liver, kidney, peas and raisins. Mollusca and shellfish are rich sources of copper, as are betel leaves and other nuts.

Recommended daily intake:
- Men and women: 1.2 mg

Iodine

Iodine is important micronutrient which is required for normal growth and development of human brain and body. It is important for the synthesis of triiodothyronine (T_3) and thyroxine (T_4). The thyroid hormones play an important role in the growth and development.

Deficiency diseases: Acne, bad circulation, confused thinking, cretinism fatigue, goiter, hormonal imbalance, menstrual difficulties miscarriages, scaly or dry skin, sterility, weight gain and weight loss, *etc.*

Overdose disease: Hyperthyroidism

Deficiency symptoms:
- Apathy
- Drowsiness
- Hair loss
- Fatigue
- Dry skin
- Increased blood fats
- Hoarseness
- Delayed reflexes
- Reduced mental clarity

Rich sources: Iodine is added to most table salt so people generally get the required amount from just one teaspoon of iodized salt. Other iodine sources include eggs, milk, sea fish and sea food, sea vegetables — such as kelp, seaweed, asparagus, *etc.* Fruits and vegetables grown in coastal regions, are other good sources of iodine.

Recommended daily intake:
- Men and women: 0.5 mg
- Females require higher iodine amounts during periods of puberty and pregnancy.

Fluoride

The fluoride mineral is one of the families of trace minerals and is one mineral that is important for teeth and bones. It occurs in the form of fluoride in nature. Fluorine is important for preventing the teeth from decaying. It is also involved in imparting stability to bone and enamel tissue. Thus, it prevents dental caries and osteoporosis.

Deficiency diseases: Cavities and weakened tooth enamel

Overdose disease: Dental fluorosis and genuvalgum (Knock knees)

Deficiency symptoms:
- Appearance of dental carries, better known as cavities
- Weakened tooth enamel
- Brittle bones

Rich sources: The chief source of fluorine is drinking water which should contain 1 part per million (ppm) of fluorine. Sea fish is also a good source of fluorine.

Selenium

Selenium is required in the diet for the proper functioning of immune system and for preventing free radical formations. It also protects against heart weakness and degeneration and is essential for the production of thyroid hormones. Selenium is found to have cancer reducing effect.

Deficiency diseases: Malabsorption, but that too is rare.

Overdose disease: Nausea, vomiting and diarrhea

Deficiency symptoms:
- Cardiovascular disease
- Nerve degeneration
- Hypothyroidism
- Arthritis
- Anemia and a dry, scaly scalp

Rich sources: Red meat, chicken, turkey, liver, fish, shellfish, dark green leafy vegetables, whole grains, eggs, onions, brazil nuts, walnuts, brewer's yeast, wheat germ, pasta, noodles, rice, cottage cheese, cheddar cheese and garlic are all good selenium sources.

Recommended daily intake:

• Men and women: 70 mg

Chromium

Chromium is needed for energy, maintains stable blood sugar levels.

Deficiency diseases: Anxiety, fatigue, glucose intolerance, inadequate metabolism of amino acids, and an increased risk of arteriosclerosis.

Overdose disease: Gastrointestinal ulcers, liver and kidney damage, and skin irritation.

Rich sources: Some of the best dietary sources of chromium include egg yolks, bread made from whole wheat, fruit juices, hard cheeses, lean beef, brewer's yeast, molasses and liver.

STUDY QUESTIONS

1. What are nutrients? How they can be classified?

2. What are the important functions of carbohydrates and proteins in the body?

3. What are lipids? State the major functions of fat in the body.

4. Explain the roles of vitamins and minerals in the body.

5. Write short notes on the following:

   a. Calcium

   b. Vitamin C

   c. Simple proteins

   d. Deficiency disorders of vitamin B_1

Importance of Dietary Fibre

Fibre is the most important component of diet which is commonly known as "roughage", is a long polymer of sugar and is classified as carbohydrate which is obtained from plants.

Fibre becomes the most important component of diet when during 1970s, Dr. Denis Burkitt, a man nicknamed the Fibre Man, and his colleagues made "the fibre hypothesis" stating the role of fibre in preventing various diseases such as heart attacks and high blood pressure (cardiovascular diseases), obesity and diabetes (metabolic disorders), intestinal problems (constipation, diverticulosis, diverticulitis, gallstones, appendicitis, hemorrhoids, polyps and colon cancer), varicose veins and blood clots. During their study they found that diseases that were common in the western cultures were not common in Africa. The only difference about the non-existence of these diseases was due to the high intake of fibre and low intake of refined carbohydrates in the African population. Burkitt in 1890 also noted the emergence of these diseases in the United States and England, after introducing a new milling technique that removed fibre from whole grain flour to produce white flour.

Burkitt again made a discovery about the beneficial impact of fibre on bowel movements and diseases. Burkitt visited a number of patients in the hospitals and noted the frequency of their bowel movements. He noted that the patient with high intakes of fibre had more frequent and bulky stools and had less illness. Burkitt proposed that fibre is beneficial for the quick stool movement through the colon thus good for gastrointestinal health.

What is Fibre?

The Institute of Medicine, states that *dietary fibre consists of nondigestible carbohydrates and lignin that are intrinsic and intact in plants and functional fibre, also called added fibre consists of isolated, nondigestible carbohydrates that have beneficial physiological effects in humans.*

According to the panel of Food and Nutrition Board, the fibre may be defined in the following ways:

- *Dietary fibre* consists of nondigestible carbohydrates and lignin that are intrinsic and intact in plants. This includes plant nonstarch polysaccharides (for example, cellulose, pectin, gums, hemicellulose and fibres contained in oat and wheat bran), oligosaccharides, lignin, and some resistant starch.
- *Functional fibre* consists of isolated, nondigestible carbohydrates that have beneficial physiological effects in humans. This includes nondigestible plant (for example, resistant starch, pectin and gums), chitin, chitosan, or commercially produced (for example, resistant starch, polydextrose, inulin, and indigestible dextrins) carbohydrates.
- *Total fibre* is the sum of *dietary fibre* and *functional fibre*.

Types of Fibre

Based on the above definitions, fibre is divided into two categories:

1. **Soluble fibre:** Soluble fibre plays an important role in absorbing the water from the intestine and thus helps in softening the stools and helps in removing the waste material through the body, quickly. The other important roles of soluble fibres in the diet are:

   i. These are helped in reducing the cholesterol in the blood.

   ii. These slows down digestion and the sudden release of energy, especially from carbohydrates into the bloodstream thus maintains the blood sugar level.

   Sources of soluble fibre: Fruits, vegetables, lentils, peas, beans, oats, barley, oatmeal, potatoes, dried fruit, soya milk and soya products are the good sources of soluble fibres.

2. **Insoluble fibre:** Insoluble fibre increases the movement of the material through the digestive tract and thus increases the bulk of the stool.

   Insoluble fibre also helps in:

   i. Promoting the growth of certain bacteria that helps in fermentation of the food material and thus makes waste material soft and bulky, which in turn passes quickly through the intestine and anus.

   ii. Preventing constipation.

   iii. Moving of wastes quickly thus no build up of toxins in the intestines takes place.

   iv. Preventing bowel cancer, constipation, irritable bowel syndrome, hemorroids and diverticulitis.

   Sources of insoluble fibre: Bran, breads, whole meal flour, brown rice, whole grain cereals, vegetables, peels of fruits, nuts and seeds are the good sources of insoluble fibres.

Roles of Fibre in Prevention of Diseases

Fibre Helps in Prevention of Gastrointestinal Disorders

Diet containing high fibre helps in preventing various gastrointestinal disorders such as constipation, diverticular disease, irritable bowel syndrome and Crohn's disease. It has been also found that dietary fibres are best for prevention and treatment of other diseases of gastrointestinal disorders such as cholelithiasis, duodenal ulcers, hemorrhoids and hiatal hernias. Dietary fibre is also helpful for the prevention of colon cancer.

Fibre in Controlling Diabetes

A high-fibre diet may help in controlling the blood sugar level. Fibre, particularly soluble fibre, can slow the absorption of sugar, thus it helps in improving blood sugar levels. A diet that includes insoluble fibre has been associated with a reduced risk of developing type 2 diabetes.

Fibre Helps in Lowering of Blood Cholesterol Level

Soluble fibre helps in lowering total blood cholesterol levels by lowering low-density lipoprotein, or "bad," cholesterol levels. The studies have shown that increased fibre in the diet can reduce blood pressure and inflammation, thus prevents heart disorders.

Fibre Helps in Preventing Obesity

High-fibre foods generally require more chewing time, which gives your body time to register when you are no longer hungry, so you are less likely to overeat. Also, a high-fibre diet tends to make a meal feel larger and linger longer, so you stay full for a greater amount of time. And high-fibre diets also tend to be less "energy dense," which means they have a fewer calories for the same volume of food.

Side Effects of High Intake of Fibre

Although fibre is the most important for the health but eating a large amount of fibre can cause various problems. A large intake of fibre may lead to flatulence, bloating, and abdominal cramps.

Large intake of fibre may also interfere with the absorption of minerals such as iron, zinc, magnesium and calcium. But, this happens rare, because high-fibre foods are typically rich in minerals.

STUDY QUESTIONS

1. What is fibre? What are various types of fibre?

2. What is the importance of fibre in our diet? Explain.

3. How fibre is important in prevention of various diseases?

4. What are the side effects of fibres?

7 Food Preservation

Food is most important for the existence of human life. Some foods are available in some seasons and not in others. Foods are obtained from various sources and thus foods fit for consumption, undergo deterioration and spoilage. So, techniques are adopted to preserve the seasonal foods for later use and also for making the food fit for consumption. The methods of food preservation are followed by men since times immemorial and now modern technology has been widely introduced in this branch, by understanding the importance of such food processing methods in human life. Hence in order to increase the shelf life foods are needed to be preserved. Preservation of food increases the shelf life of foods and thus ultimately ensures its supply during times of scarcity and natural drought.

DEFINITIONS

Food preservation can be defined *as the science that deals with the process of prevention of decay or spoilage of food thus allowing it to be stored in a fit condition for future use.*

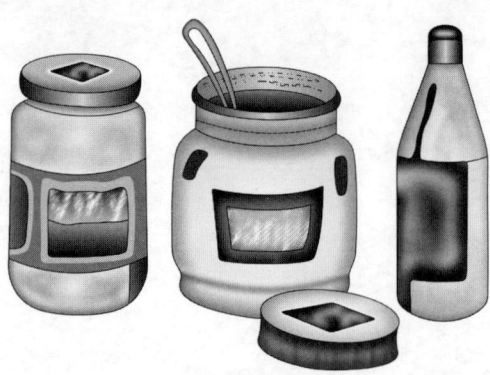

Food preservation has also been defined as, "the science which deals with the process of prevention of decay or spoilage of food thus allowing it to be stored in a fit condition for future use."

It has also been described as the state in which any food may be retained over a period of time without:

1. being contaminated by pathogenic organisms or chemicals.
2. losing optimum qualities of color, texture, flavor and nutritive value.

Food preservation is *a process by which certain foods like fruits and vegetables are prevented from getting spoilt for a long period of time. The color, taste and nutritive value of the food is also preserved.*

Hence, it is clear from the definitions that the preserved food should *retain its color and taste* and the color and taste of food which are present at the time of preservation should not change.

Besides colour and taste, a well preserved food should *not change texture.*

Importance of Food Preservation: Food preservation is important because:

1. Food preservation is important for increasing the self-life of food which ultimately results in increase of supply of food. So many perishable foods can be preserved for a long time.
2. Food preservation is a best way of making the seasonal food available throughout the year.
3. It is a good way of adding variety to the diet.

4. Saving time by reducing preparation time and energy, as the food has already been partially processed.

5. Food preservation will lead to stabilization of food prices, as there is less scope of shortage of supply to demand.

6. It will result in decreasing wastage of food by preventing decay or spoilage of food.

7. Improving the nutritional status of the population. Preserved foods help people to bring a variety in the diet, thereby decreasing nutritional inadequacies.

FOOD SPOILAGE

Food spoilage is a state in which food quality becomes defective and it gets deteriorated. Deterioration or spoilage starts from the time when food is harvested, slaughtered or manufactured and results in undesirable changes in the physical and chemical characteristics of food.

Food is said to be spoilt if there is rotting, i.e. bad smell, fermentation, that is, bubbles/gas in the food or mold, that is, spongy growth on the foodstuff. Formation of soft spots or soft brown spots on fruits and vegetables is also food spoilage.

Hence, it is cleared that any change in the quality is a sign of food spoilage and the important causes of food spoilage are the presence of microorganisms, enzymes (present in foods), insects, worms and rats. These can be discussed as:

1. **Presence of microorganisms:** Microorganisms are very small organisms which cannot be easily seen. These spoil food items when these are found suitable conditions for their growth. Like all living beings microorganisms require air, moisture, right temperature and food to grow and multiply. The bruised skin of fruits and vegetables is a suitable way for development of microorganisms. Foods with low salt, sugar or acid content also results in spoilage of foods. Thus, it is necessary that the food must be well washed and cleaned before use.

2. **Presence of enzymes:** Enzymes are chemical substances found in all plants and animals and these help in ripening of fruits and vegetables. A raw green mango after a few days becomes sweet in taste and yellow in colour due to the enzymes action. After ripening, when the foods are left, then these are became softer, and black spots are also developed. All this will result the food to smell bad. This is due to continued action of enzymes and all this will lead to deterioration of food items.

3. **Insects, worms and rats:** In the grains and pulses, small insects develop and these insects eat the food grains. They make small holes in the grain and at times convert the grain to a fine powder. The food grains thus become unfit for human consumption.

Sometimes the rats may lead to the deterioration of foods and they spoil the food by their excreta and thus the food becomes unfit for consumption.

PRINCIPLES OF FOOD PRESERVATION

In order to prevent the food from spoilage, it is necessary that the food items should be preserved. A good method of food preservation is one that slows down or prevents altogether the action of the agents of spoilage. Also, during the process of food preservation, the food should not be damaged.

In order to achieve these aspects, the basic principles should be applied. These are:

1. Prevention or delay of microbial decomposition.
   a. by keeping out microorganisms (asepsis)
   b. by removal of microorganisms (e.g. filtration)
   c. by hindering the growth and activity of microorganisms. (e.g. refrigeration, dehydration, addition of chemical preservatives.)
   d. by killing microorganisms (e.g. boiling, irradiation.)

2. Prevention or delay of self-decomposition of food.

a. by destruction or inactivation of enzymes, e.g. by blanching. The steaming or boiling of fruits or vegetables in water for a few minutes to inactivate natural enzymes and facilitates removal of skin is known as blanching.

b. by prevention or delay of purely chemical reactions, e.g. prevention of oxidation by the use of antioxidants.

3. Prevention of damage caused by insects, animals and mechanical causes.

METHODS OF FOOD PRESERVATION

A perusal of the history of food preservation reveals that food preservation had its beginning from time immemorial and could be traced to nearly a thousand years ago. Salting of meat, fish and vegetables was the oldest method of preservation and could be traced back to the ancient Egypt and Greek civilizations. Pickling in salt and vinegar, sun-drying and preservation of fruits and vegetables in sugar and honey were among the other methods used. Storage of food in frozen conditions was also practiced for centuries in places where freezing temperatures were recorded. All methods used for food preservation are based on preventing or retarding the cause of spoilage. When growth of microorganism is only retarded, preservation is temporary. When spoilage organisms are completely destroyed, a more permanent preservation is achieved.

Use of Low and High Temperatures

Use of low temperatures: The growth of the microorganisms and the enzymatic reactions in the foods can be retarded by storing the food at low temperatures. The lower the temperature, longer is the duration for which food can be preserved. The food is thus prevented from spoilage.

The low temperatures employed can be:

1. Cellar storage temperature (about 15 °C)

2. Refrigerator or chilling temperature (0 to 5 °C).

3. Freezing temperature (–18 to –40 °C).

Cellar Storage Temperatures (about 15 °C)

Cellars are the underground rooms, where surplus food is stored in many villages. The temperatures in cellars are usually not much below that of the outside air and are seldom lower than 15 °C. Decomposition is slowed down considerably. Root crops, potatoes, onions, apples and similar foods can be stored for limited periods during the winter months.

Refrigerator or Chilling Temperature (0 to 5 °C)

Chilling (refrigerator) temperatures are obtained and maintained by means of ice or mechanical refrigeration. Fruits and vegetables, meats, poultry, fresh milk and milk products, fish and eggs can be preserved from two days to a week when held at this temperature.

In addition to the foods mentioned above, foods prepared for serving or left-overs may also be stored in the household refrigerator. The best storage temperature for many foods, for example, eggs, is slightly above 0 °C.

The optimum temperature of storage varies with the product and is fairly specific for any given food. Besides temperature, the relative humidity and the composition of the atmosphere can affect the preservation of the food.

Commercial cold storages with proper ventilation and automatic control of temperatures are now used throughout the country (mostly in cities) for the storage of semiperishable products such as potatoes and apples. This has made such foods available throughout the year and has also stabilized their prices in these cities.

Low temperatures chiefly inhibit the growth of microorganisms although freezing may result in the destruction of some microorganisms.

Freezing Temperature

Freezing is another medium for the prevention of microorganism. The chief preservative effect of freezing lies in the inability of microorganisms to grow at freezing temperature. Freezing may preserve foods for long periods of time and also the quality of the food is retained.

In vegetables, enzyme action may still produce undesirable effects on flavor and texture during freezing. The enzymes, therefore, must be destroyed by heating before the vegetables are frozen.

Slow freezing process

This method is also known as sharp freezing. In this method, the foods are placed in refrigerated cabinets at temperatures ranging from –4 to –29 °C. This method is adopted in home-freezers. Freezing may require from 3 to 72 hours under such conditions.

Quick freezing process

The quick freezing process employs the lower temperature that is around –32 to –40 °C. At this temperature fine crystals are formed rapidly and also the time of freezing is greatly reduced over that required in sharp freezing. The fine crystals formed by quick freezing have a lesser effect on breaking up plant and animal cells than do methods of slow freezing that produce coarser ice crystals. The advantage of this method is that, large quantity of food can be frozen in a short period of time.

Dehydro-freezing

Dehydro-freezing of fruits and vegetables consists of drying the food about 50 percent of its original weight and volume and then freezing the food to preserve it.

The quality of dehydro-frozen fruits and vegetables is equal to that of fruits and vegetables frozen without preliminary drying.

The cost in packing, freezing, storing and shipping of such foods is less because of the reduction in weight and volume of foods during dehydro-freezing.

The rapid growth of bacteria occurs in the temperature zone of 60 –120 °F.

Use of Heat or High Temperatures

The destruction of microorganisms by heat is due to the coagulation of the protoplasm. The temperature and time used in heat processing a food depend upon the nature of the food and what other methods are combined with heat.

The various degrees of heating used in preservation of food can be classified into three types:

a. Pasteurization,

b. Heating up to 100 °C or 212 °F and

c. Heating above 100 °C.

a. *Pasteurization*: Around 1860, Louis Pasteur discovered that microbes were the main cause of spoilage and introduced a heat treatment known as pasteurization. Pasteurization is defined as partial sterilization of foods at a temperature that destroys harmful microorganisms without major changes in the chemistry of the food. The method employed in pasteurization required 100 °C for preservation of foods. The time and temperature used in the pasteurization process depend upon the product treated and the method used. In pasteurization, most of the spoilage organisms are killed but a few survive and hence must be inhibited by low temperatures or some other methods, if spoilage is to be prevented. Milk is nowadays is pasteurized by the temperature that inhibits the growth of the microorganisms that may have survived. Beer, fruit juices and aerated drinks are preserved by this method.

There are two methods of pasteurization:

1. *Flash method*: This method is also known as high temperature short time method, that is, a high temperature for a short time is used.

2. *Holder method*: Also called low-temperature time method that is a lower temperature for a longer time is used.

There are slight variations in the time and temperature used for pasteurizing different foods, like milk, cream, ice cream mix and wines.

b. *Heating up to a temperature of about 100 °C*: At this temperature, mostly cooking is done. This temperature can be obtained by boiling any liquid food, by immersing a container in boiling water or by exposure to steam. Before the use of pressure cookers and autoclaves, canning is done at 100 °C and this kills all bacteria except spores.

c. *Heating above 100 °C (212 °F)*: Temperatures above 100 °C are obtained by means of steam under pressure as in a pressure cooker or autoclave. Sterilization of foods can be brought about at 121 °C for 15 minutes under moist conditions.

Canning

The technique of canning was discovered by Nicholas Appert in 1810. This is a standard technique of preserving foods in sealed containers by using high temperature. In the process of canning, the foods are first cleaned and then they are blanched to soften the fibrous plant tissues, and to inhibit the action of enzymes. After blanching gases are expelled by passing the open can containing the food through an exhaust box in which hot water or steam is used to expand the food and expel air and other gases from the contents and the head space area of the can. After the gases are expelled, the can is immediately sealed, heat processed and cooled.

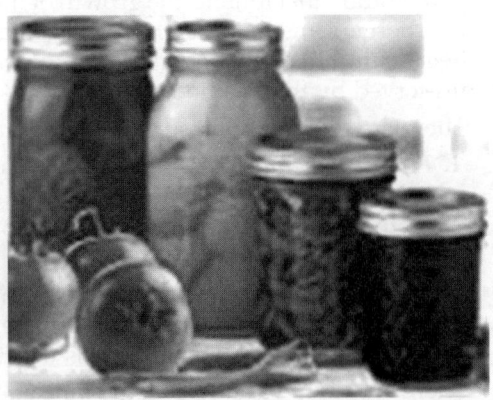

Drying

Moisture is one of the important conditions in which microorganisms can easily grow. Due to presence of moisture, microorganisms grow and food is spoiled. Hence, food items are dried to prevent the growth of microorganisms. The food items are thus exposed to sunlight or subjected to dehydration, so that the moisture in the food is removed and the concentration of water is brought below a certain level. This prevents the growth of microorganisms and thereby spoilage of food. Food preservation by drying is one of the oldest methods practiced from ancient times. This method consists of exposing food to sunlight and air until the product is dry.

Treatment of foods before drying
- The food items are selected according to their size and shape.
- They are then washed thoroughly, if needed.
- Foods such as fruits and vegetables are peeled by hand, machine or abrasion.
- They are then divided into halves or cut into slices, shreds or cubes.
- Blanching or scalding of vegetables and some fruits like apricots and peaches should be done.

Methods of Drying
Sun drying: In this method food items are sun dried by exposing them to direct sunlight. Sun drying is a slow process, thus is time taking. Many Indian foods are preserved by sun drying. Papads and mango powder are made using this principle. Vegetables like potatoes and chilies and fruits like jackfruit and mango are preserved by this method. Fish and meat are also sun dried.

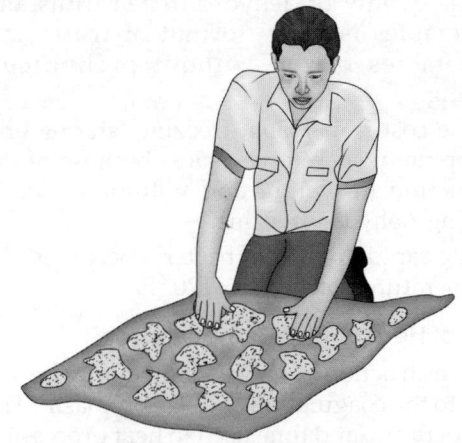

Drying by mechanical driers: Mechanical drying is an artificial drying process which involves the passage of heated air with controlled relative humidity over the food to be dried or the passage of the food through such air. Fruits, vegetables, nuts, fish and meat can be successfully preserved by this method. In the dehydration process, artificial drying methods (e.g. spray drier) are used for drying foods. Although, it is expensive when compared to natural sun-drying procedures, it is very advantageous because the temperature and relative humidity can be manipulated.

Spray drying: Milk and egg are dried to a powder in spray driers in which the liquid is atomized and sprayed into a hot air stream for almost instant drying.

Foam mat drying: Foam mat drying is a commercial way in which orange and tomato juices are dried. In this process a small amount of edible foam stabilizer such as monoglycerides or a modified soyabean protein with methyl cellulose is added to the liquid and stiff foam is produced by whipping. The foam is spread in a thin layer and dried in a stream of hot air. The product separates easily into small particles on cooling.

Drying by osmosis: In osmotic dehydration of fruits, the method involves the partial dehydration of fruits by osmosis in a concentrated sugar solution or syrup. In this case, the moisture is drawn out from all cell tissues. Drying also results when fish is heavily salted. The water is then bound with the solute, making it unavailable to the microorganisms.

Freeze drying: Removal of water from a product while it is frozen by sublimations is called freeze drying.

Factors to be considered in drying foods:

- The temperature employed, which will vary with the food and the method of drying.
- The relative humidity of the air. It is usually higher at the start of drying than later.
- The velocity of the air.
- The duration of drying.

Use of High Concentration of Sugar and Salt

Sugar and salt aid in the preservation of products in which it is used due to their ability to bind water and make it unavailable for microbial growth. Salt is an effective preservative because it also ionizes to yield chlorine ion, which is harmful to organisms and reduces the solubility of oxygen in moisture, which are essential for the growth, and multiplication of microorganisms. Jams, jellies and fruit juices are the important class of fruit products preserved using high concentration of sugar. Pickles are preserved using high concentration of salt.

Jam: Jams are prepared by boiling fruit pulp with sufficient amount of sugar to a reasonably thick consistency, firm enough to hold the fruit tissue in position. In preparing jam, the fruit is crushed or finely cut and measured the quantity of sugar and preservatives are added so that when cooked, the mass is fairly uniform throughout. Jams can be prepared from all varieties of pulpy fruits such as grapes, mango, sapota, banana, guava, *etc.*

Jelly: Jellies are prepared by boiling fruits in water. The extract obtained is strained and measured the quantity of sugar is added to it. The mixture is then boiled to a stage at which it will set to a clear gel. A perfect jelly should be transparent, well set, but not too stiff and should have the original flavor of the fruit. It should retain its shape when removed from the mould. Usually, fruits such as guava, pineapple, apple, grape and a mixture of fruits rich in pectin can be used for the preparation of jellies.

Fruit juices: Fruit beverages are prepared from different fruits such as apple, mango, grapes, lime, pineapple, oranges and in different forms such as pure juices, crushes, squashes and cordials. The ratios of sugar and fruit juice in the preparation of various beverages are as follows:

Crushes— 25% fruit juice and 55% sugar.
Squashes— 25% fruit juice and 45% sugar.
Cordial— clarified juice 1 liter and 250 gm sugar.

In the preparation of fruit juices, citric acid is usually added to clarify the sugar syrup. Preservatives such as sodium benzoate are added to tomato and grape juices while potassium meta-bisulfite (KMS) is added to all other fruit beverages.

Pickling: Pickling is a home practice which is done to add taste in diet. The preservation of fruits and vegetables in common salt, vinegar, oil and spices are referred to as pickling. Salt binds the moisture in the food and thereby prevents the growth of microorganisms.

The layer of oil that floats on the top of pickles prevents the entry and growth of microorganisms like moulds and yeast. Spices like turmeric, pepper, chilli powder and asafoetida retard the growth of bacteria. Vinegar lowers the pH of the product, thereby providing an unfavorable acidic environment for microbial growth. Mango, lime, ginger, garlic, tomato, chilli, mixed vegetables such as beans, carrot, cauliflower and peas are used widely in the preparation of pickles.

Use of Chemical Preservatives

Preservatives are defined as chemical agents who serve to retard, hinder or mask the undesirable changes in food. These changes may be caused by microorganisms, by enzymes of food or by purely chemical reactions. Certain chemicals when added in small quantities can hinder undesirable chemical reaction in food by:

1. interfering with the cell membrane of the microorganism, their enzyme activity or their genetic mechanism.
2. acting as antioxidants.

Preservatives must be added in limited amount as higher amount may lead to health hazard. Benzoic acid in the form of its sodium salt is an effective inhibitor of moulds and is used extensively for the preservation of jams and jellies.

Some of the other chemical preservatives used are:

1. Potassium metabisulfite
2. Sorbic acid
3. Calcium propionate
4. Sodium benzoate

The development of off-flavors (rancidity) in edible oils is prevented by the use of butylated hydroxy anisole (BHA), butylated hydroxy toluene (BHT), lecithin, are some of the approved antioxidants.

Radiation

Radiant energy can be used to preserve food. Gamma rays and beta particles produced by special electronic machines are sources of energy used to preserve food. These waves penetrate throughout the food. As the waves and particles pass through the food, they collide with molecules in the food and in microorganisms. These result in chemical alterations. The goal of irradiation is to kill the microorganism and inactivate the enzymes without altering the food. Changes in the food are minimized, if it is done in a vacuum, and if ascorbic acid is present. Berries and meat are preserved in this way.

STUDY QUESTIONS

1. Define preservation. What are the principles of food preservation?
2. What are the causes of food spoilage?
3. How does salt and sugar lend themselves as preservatives?
4. Differentiate jams and jellies.
5. What are the functions of the ingredients used in pickling?
6. Write a note on chemical preservatives and its use.
7. How do low temperature procedures prevent spoilage? Discuss the methods.
8. Give a brief account on any four techniques employed in food preservation.
9. Explain the use of high temperature in food preservation.
10. Define canning. Explain the steps in canning.
11. Give a detailed account on drying as a method of preservation. Write a note on the different types of drying.

8 Food Adulteration

Adulteration is the most common harmful practice mainly done by the traders either for financial gain or due to carelessness and lack in proper hygienic condition of processing, storing, transportation and marketing. This ultimately results that the consumer is either cheated or often become victim of diseases. When the price of the food product is higher than the price which the consumer is prepared to pay, seller is compelled to supply a food product of inferior quality, and thus adulteration occurs. Such types of adulteration are quite common in developing countries or backward countries. However, adequate precautions taken by the consumer at the time of purchase of such product can make him alert to avoid procurement of such food. It is equally important for the consumer to know the common adulterants and their effect on health.

DEFINITION

Adulteration usually refers to mixing other matter of an inferior and sometimes harmful quality with food or drink intended to be sold.

It is also defined as the process by which the quality or the nature of a given substance is reduced through:

 i. the addition of a foreign or an inferior substance, for example, the addition of water to milk.
 ii. the removal of a vital element, for example, the removal of fat from milk.

Adulteration of food is harmful for health, and affects the physiological functions of the consumers due to either addition of a deleterious substance or the removal of a vital component.

Problems due to adulteration: Food adulteration, apart from cheating the consumers, often results in disorders or diseases. Some of the foods commonly adulterated in India and problems are as follows:

Pulses like masoor, black gram and channa are mixed with kesari dhal. Consumption of kesari dhal for a long time causes lathyrism which results in paralysis of the lower limbs.

Roasted tamarind and date seeds are ground and adulterated with coffee powder.

Edible oils and fats are adulterated with cheap edible and nonedible oils. Argemone seeds resemble mustard and are used to mix with mustard seeds. Argemone oil itself extracted from the seeds, is used to adulterate oil such as coconut, sesame and groundnut. Argemone oil is poisonous and its use results in dropsy in human beings. Fats and oils are also adulterated with petroleum products causing gastrointestinal disturbances.

The most frequently used food adulterant in India is colouring matter. Colour is used in many foods such as milk products, confectionary, soft drinks, alcoholic beverages, tea and spices. Colours are also added to foods such as egg preparations, bakery products, fruit products and others. More than 70 percent of the colours containing marketed samples of foods are found to contain no permitted colourants like lead chromate and coal tar dyes. Use of foods containing nonpermitted colourants result in various health hazards.

Table 8.1: Injurious adulterants/contaminants in foods and their health effects

S.No.	Adulterant	Foods commonly involved	Diseases or health effects
1.	Argemone seeds Argemone oil	Mustard seeds Edible oils and fats	Epidemic dropsy, glaucoma, cardiac arrest
2.	Artificially coloured foreign seeds	As a substitute for cumin seed, poppy seed, black pepper	Injurious to health
3.	Foreign leaves or exhausted tea leaves, saw dust artificially coloured	Tea	Injurious to health, cancer
5.	Rancid oil	Oils	Destroys vitamin A and E
6.	Sand, marble chips, stones,	Food grains, pulses, *etc.*	Damage digestive tract
7.	*Lathyrus sativus*	Khesari dal alone or mixed in other pulses	Lathyrism (crippling spastic paraplegia)

Types of Adulterants: Adulterants may be of two types:

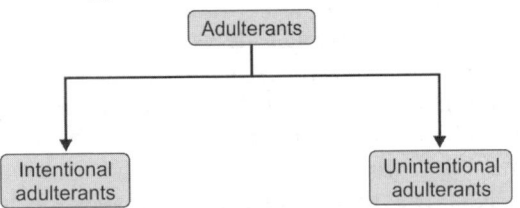

Intentional adulteration: Intentional adulteration is a willful act on the part of the adulterator intended to increase the margin of profit. Intentional adulterants are sand, marble chips, stones, mud, chalk powder, water, mineral oil and coal tar dyes. These adulterants cause harmful effects on the body.

Incidental or unintentional adulteration: Incidental adulteration is usually due to ignorance, negligence or lack of proper facilities.

Incidental Adulteration

1. **Contamination of foods with harmful microorganisms:** The foods which are sold near the sewage or those which are washed by using the sewage water are likely to be contaminated with harmful microorganisms. These microorganisms are generally destroyed during cooking or processing of food. Recent studies have shown that food grains, legumes and oil seeds when stored in humid atmosphere are infected by pathogenic fungus which can cause serious illness.

2. **Metallic contamination:** The chemicals such as arsenic, lead or mercury get accumulated in the body, which can be harmful. Lead is a toxic element and contamination of food with lead can cause toxicity in the body. Lead brings about pathological changes in the kidneys, liver and arteries. For example, turmeric is coated with lead chromate. The common signs of lead poisoning are nausea, abdominal pain, anemia, insomnia, muscular paralysis and brain damage. Fish caught from water contaminated with mercuric salts contain large amounts of mercury. The toxic elements which are toxic in small doses are cadmium, arsenic, antimony and cobalt.

Table 8.2: Toxic effects of some chemicals and metals and their harmful effects on health

S. No.	Chemicals and metals	Foods commonly involved	Diseases or health effects
1.	Lead chromate	Turmeric whole and powdered, mixed spices	Anemia, abortion, paralysis, brain damage
2.	Methanol	Alcoholic liquors	Blurred vision, blindness, death
3.	Arsenic	Fruits such as apples sprayed over with lead arsenate	Dizziness, chills, cramps, paralysis, death

Contd.

Table 8.2: Toxic effects of some chemicals and metals and their harmful effects on health *(Contd.)*

S. No.	Chemicals and metals	Foods commonly involved	Diseases or health effects
4.	Barium	Foods contaminated by rat poisons (Barium carbonate)	Violent peristalsis, arterial hypertension, muscular twitching, convulsions, cardiac disturbances
5.	Cadmium	Fruit juices, soft drinks, *etc.* in contact with cadmium plated vessels or equipment. Cadmium contaminated water and shellfish	Itai-itai (ouch-ouch) disease, increased salivation, acute gastritis, liver and kidney damage, prostrate cancer
6.	Cobalt	Water, liquors	Cardiac insufficiency and mycocardial failure
7.	Lead	Water, natural and processed food	Lead poisoning (foot-drop, insomnia, anemia, constipation, mental retardation, brain damage)
8.	Copper	Food	Vomiting, diarrhea
9.	Tin	Food	Colic, vomiting
10.	Zinc	Food	Colic, vomiting
11.	Mercury	Mercury fungicide treated seed grains or mercury contaminated fish	Brain damage, paralysis, death
12.	Mineral oil (white oil, petroleum fractions)	Edible oils and fats, black pepper	Cancer

3. **Other incidental adulterants:** Pests such as rats, rodents and insects introduce into the food a high degree of filth in the form of excreta, bodily secretions and spoilage microorganisms. The chemicals like DDT which are sprayed on the plants, when ingested, are absorbed by the small intestine and cause toxicity. The toxins usually pile up in the fatty tissues of such vital organs as the thyroid, heart, kidney, liver, mammary gland and damage these organs. They can be transferred from the umbilical cord blood to the growing foetus or through breast milk to infants. In children the disease, apart from crippling them, inhibits their growth.

The health department sprays pesticides to control malaria causing mosquitoes. Residues remain long after spraying pesticides. Cattle fodder and chicken feed are affected. Groundwater is poisoned. Meat, fish, milk and egg are affected by toxins. To protect the grains in the store spraying is done to prevent fungus and rodents. This leads to an increase in the residue levels in foodstuffs. Sellers dip vegetables in pesticides to make them look fresh as well as to preserve them. Oils and sweets are adulterated with prohibited substances. Washing and cooking rarely destroys toxic residues. When ingested, pesticides are absorbed by small intestine. The fatty tissues distributed throughout the body store these pesticides. These can damage vital organs like the heart, brain, kidney and liver.

Prevention of incidental poisoning: This can be prevented by:
- Regular market surveys to warn people on the dangerous build-up of toxins in food.
- Stepping up the integrated pest management programme to teach farmers to use pesticides judiciously. No spraying should be done a week before harvest.
- Using safer pesticides
- Washing vegetables thoroughly before cooking.

New adulterants: The newer adulterants include the legumes such as imported toxic lentils marketed as local lentils, veterinary drug residues in milk, flours made from mouldy wheat, animal fat in bakery products and industrial contamination in vanaspati. Ginger is used widely in culinary practice in India in the fresh or dry form. Dry ginger is often coated with blue coloured dye ultramarine blue to prevent insect infestation. It is an inorganic pigment used as laundry whitener.

4. **Packaging hazards:** Today the foods are sold in packets and the material used for packaging are polyethylene, polyvinyl chloride and allied compounds are used. This method of packaging is very convenient, but it produces noxious thermal breakdown products which are injurious to health. Further, temperatures used for heat sealing or sterilization results in the formation of toxic residues. It has been observed that in foods like pickles, the acid

and oil could attack the plastic packaging material and create a health hazard. To avoid such incidences, it is essential that only food grade plastic packaging materials should be used for packaging foods.

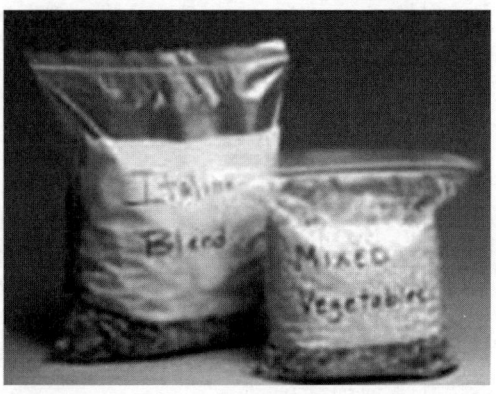

DETECTION OF FOOD ADULTERANTS

In order to detect the presence of adulterants in the food some tests are used. The food articles containing the adulterants and the specific test done to know about the presence of adulterants are shown in Table 8.3.

Table 8.3: Specific test to know about the presence of adulterants

S.No.	Food article	Adulteration	Test
1.	Vegetable oil	Castor oil	Take 1 ml of oil in a clean dry test tube. Add 10 ml of acidified petroleum ether. Shake vigorously for 2 minutes. Add 1 drop of ammonium molybdate reagent. The formation of turbidity indicates presence of castor oil in the sample.
		Argemone oil	Add 5 ml, conc. HNO_3 to 5 ml sample. Shake carefully. Allow to separate yellow, orange yellow, crimson colour in the lower acid layer indicates adulteration.
2.	Ghee	Mashed potato, sweet potato, *etc.*	Boil 5 ml of the sample in a test tube. Cool and add a drop of iodine solution. Blue colour indicates presence of Starch. Colour disappears on boiling and reappears on cooling.
		Vanaspati	Take 5 ml of the sample in a test tube. Add 5 ml of hydrochloric acid and 0.4 ml of 2% furfural solution or sugar crystals. Insert the glass stopper and shake for 2 minutes. Development of a pink or red colour indicates presence of vanaspati in ghee.
		Rancid stuff (old ghee)	Take one teaspoon of melted sample and 5 ml of HCl in a stoppered glass tube. Shake vigorously for 30 seconds. Add 5 ml of 0.1% of ether solution of phloroglucinol. Restopper & shake for 30 seconds and allow to stand for 10 minutes. A pink or red colour in the lower (acid layer) indicates rancidity.
		Synthetic colouring matter	Pour 2 gm of filtered fat dissolved in ether. Divide into 2 portions. Add 1 ml of HCl to one tube. Add 1 ml of 10% NaOH to the other tube. Shake well and allow to stand. Presence of pink colour in acidic solution or yellow colour in alkaline solution indicates added colouring matter.

Contd.

Table 8.3: Specific test to know about the presence of adulterants (*Contd.*)

S.No.	Food article	Adulteration	Test
3.	Honey	Invert sugar/jaggery	1. Fiehe's Test: Add 5 ml of solvent ether to 5 ml of honey. Shake well and decant the ether layer in a petri dish. Evaporate completely by blowing the ether layer. Add 2 to 3 ml of resorcinol (1 gm of resorcinol resublimed in 5 ml of conc. HCl.). Appearance of cherry red colour indicates presence of sugar/jaggery.
			2. Aniline chloride test: Take 5 ml of honey in a porcelain dish. Add aniline chloride solution (3 ml of Aniline and 7 ml of 1:3 HCl) and stir well. Orange red colour indicates presence of sugar.
4.	Pulses/besan	Kesari dal (Lathyrus sativus)	Add 50 ml of dil. HCl to a small quantity of dal and keep on simmering water for about 15 minutes. The pink colour, if developed, indicates the presence of Kesari dal.
5.	Pulses	Metanil yellow (dye)	Add conc. HCl to a small quantity of dal in a little amount of water. Immediate development of pink colour indicates the presence of metanil yellow and similar colour dyes.
		Lead chromate	Shake 5 gm of pulse with 5 ml of water and add a few drops of HCl. Pink colour indicates lead chromate.
6.	Bajra	Ergot infested Bajra	Swollen and black ergot infested grains will turn light in weight and will float also in water
7.	Wheat flour	Excessive sand and dirt	Shake a little quantity of sample with about 10 ml of carbon tetra chloride and allow to stand. Grit and sandy matter will collect at the bottom.
		Excessive bran	Sprinkle on water surface. Bran will float on the surface.
8.	Common spices like turmeric, chilly, curry powder, *etc.*	Chalk powder	Shake sample with dil.HCl. Effervescence indicates chalk.
		Colour	Extract the sample with petroleum ether and add 13 N H_2SO_4 to the extract. Appearance of red colour (which persists even upon adding little distilled water) indicates the presence of added colours. However, if the colour disappears upon adding distilled water, the sample is not adulterated.
9.	Black pepper	Papaya seeds/light berries, *etc.*	Pour the seeds in a beaker containing carbon tetrachloride. Black papaya seeds float on the top while the pure black pepper seeds settle down.
10.	Spices (Ground)	Powdered bran and sawdust	Sprinkle on water surface. Powdered bran and sawdust float on the surface.
11.	Coriander powder	Dung powder	Soak in water. Dung will float and can be easily detected by its foul smell.
		Common salt	To 5 ml of sample, add a few drops of silver nitrate. White precipitate indicates adulteration.
12.	Chillies	Brick powder grit, sand, dirt, filth, *etc.*	Pour the sample in a beaker containing a mixture of chloroform and carbon tetrachloride. Brick powder and grit will settle at the bottom.
13.	Badi elaichi seeds	Choti elaichi seeds	Separate out the seeds by physical examination. The seeds of badi elaichi have nearly plain surface without wrinkles or streaks while seeds of cardamom have pitted or wrinkled ends.
14.	Turmeric powder	Starch of maize, wheat, tapioca, rice	A microscopic study reveals that only pure turmeric is yellow coloured, big in size and has an angular structure. While foreign/added starches are colourless and small in size as compared to pure turmeric starch.

Contd.

Table 8.3: Specific test to know about the presence of adulterants *(Contd.)*

S.No.	Food article	Adulteration	Test
15.	Turmeric	Lead chromate	Ash the sample. Dissolve it in 1:7 sulphuric acid (H_2SO_4) and filter. Add 1 or 2 drops of 0.1% diphenylcarbazide. A pink colour indicates presence of lead chromate.
		Metanil yellow	Add a few drops of conc. hydrochloric acid (HCl) to sample. Instant appearance of violet colour, which disappears on dilution with water, indicates pure turmeric. If colour persists, metanil yellow is present.
16.	Cumin seeds (Black jeera)	Grass seeds coloured with charcoal dust	Rub the cumin seeds on palms. If palms turn black, adulteration is indicated.
17.	Asafoetida (Heeng)	Soap stone, other earthy matter	Shake a little quantity of powdered sample with water. Soap stone or other earthy matter will settle at the bottom.
		Chalk	Shake sample with carbon tetrachloride (CCl_4). Asafoetida will settle down. Decant the top layer and add dil. HCl to the residue. Effervescence shows presence of chalk.
18.	Food grains	Hidden insect infestation	Take a filter paper impregnated with ninhydrin (1% in alcohol). Put some grains on it and then fold the filter paper and crush the grains with hammer. Spots of bluish purple colour indicate presence of hidden insects infestation.

FOOD LAWS AND STANDARDS— PFA, AGMARK, BIS, FPO, CONSUMER PROTECTION ACT

In order to meet the country's health requirements and to meet the market access, Government of India has promulgated many laws and standards. These laws ensure the safety and suitability of food for consumers.

Food Laws and Standards

Food Safety and Standards Act: The Indian parliament has recently passed the Food Safety and Standards Act, 2006, that overrides all other food related laws. It covers eight laws:

- Prevention of Food Adulteration Act, 1954
- Fruit Products Order, 1955
- Meat Products Order, 1973
- Vegetable Oil Products (Control) Order, 1947
- Edible Oil Packaging (Regulation) Order, 1998
- Solvent Extracted Oil, Deoiled Meal and Edible Flour (Control) Order, 1967
- Milk and Milk Products Order, 1992
- Essential Commodities Act, 1955 (relating to food)

The Act establishes a new national regulatory body and the Food Safety and Standards Authority of India, develop science based standards for food and regulate and monitor the manufacture, processing, storage, distribution, sale and import of food so as to ensure the availability of safe and wholesome food for human consumption.

1. **Prevention of Food Adulteration Act (PFA, 1954):** One of the early Acts to be promulgated was the Prevention of Food Adulteration Act of 1954, which was in force since June 1, 1955. The objective of this act was to ensure that food articles sold to the consumers are pure and wholesome. The act prohibits the manufacture, sale and distribution of not only adulterated foods but also foods contaminated with microorganisms and toxicants. PFA specifies microbial safety standards for pasteurized milk, milk powder, skimmed milk powder, infant milk food, tomato sauce, jam, malted milk food and aflatoxin levels for groundnut.

The PFA standards and regulations apply equally to domestic and imported products and cover various aspects of food processing and distribution. These include food colours, preservatives, pesticide residues, packaging and labelling and regulation of sales. 'A central committee for food standards' has been constituted under the Act and has been charged with the function of advising the central government on matters relating to the food standards. The state government sets up food testing laboratory and appoints Public Analysts with adequate staff to report on suspected foods.

2. **Fruit Products Order (1955):** The fruit and vegetable processing sector is regulated by the Fruit Products Order (FPO), 1955, which is administered by the department of food processing industries. The FPO contains specifications and quality control requirements regarding the production and marketing of processed fruits and vegetables, sweetened aerated water, vinegar and synthetic syrups. Packaging fruits and vegetables of a standard below the minimum prescribed standards is an offence, punishable by law. All processing units are required to obtain a licence under the FPO, and periodic inspections are carried out. Processed fruits and vegetable products imported into the country must meet the FPO standards.

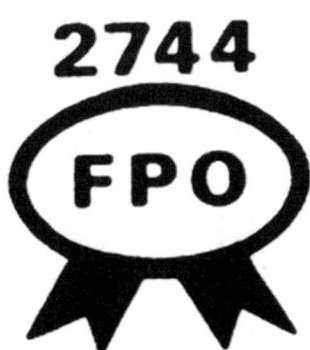

3. **Meat Products Order (1973):** The regulations made under the act covers the meat products and:
    • Specifies sanitation and hygienic requirements for slaughter houses and manufacture of meat products.
    • Contains packing, marking and labelling provisions for containers of meat products.

• Defines the permissible quantity of heavy metals, preservatives and insecticide residues in meat products.
• Prevents the use of harmful substances in meat food products.

The Directorate of marketing and inspection at the ministry of agriculture is the regulatory authority for the order, which is equally applicable to domestic processors and importers of meat products.

4. **Livestock Importation Act (1898):** India has established procedures for the importation of livestock under the Livestock Importation Act, 1898. Under the regulations, the import of meat products, eggs and egg powder and milk products require a sanitary import permit from the Department of Animal Husbandry, Dairying and Fisheries at the Ministry of Agriculture.

5. **Milk and Milk Products Order (1992):** Under milk and milk products order the production and distribution or supply of milk products is controlled by the Milk and Milk Products Order, 1992. The order sets sanitary requirements for dairies, machinery and premises and includes quality control, certification, packing, marketing and labeling standards for milk and milk products. Standards specified in the order also apply to imported products.

6. **Essential Commodities Act (1955):** The Act is mainly meant for regulating the manufacture, commerce and distribution of essential commodities including food to the public at reasonable price.

7. **Cold Storage Order (1980):** The cold storage order, 1980, promulgated under the Essential Commodities Act, 1955, has the objective of earning hygienic and proper refrigeration conditions in a cold store regulating the growth of cold storage industry and rendering technical guidance for the scientific preservation of foodstuffs in a cold store and prevent exploitation of farmers by cold store owners. Agricultural marketing advisor to the Government of India is the licensing officer under this.

8. **Weights and Measures Act (1976):** Standards for weights and measures are administered by the Ministry of Consumer Affairs, Food and Public Distribution under the Standards of Weights and Measures Act, 1976 and related rules and notification. All weights or measures must be recorded in metric units and certain commodities can only be packed in specified quantities (weight, measure or number). These include baby and weaning foods, biscuits, bread, butter, coffee, tea, vegetable oils, milk powder, and wheat and rice flour.

Bureau of Indian Standards (BIS)

The Bureau of Indian Standards operates certification mark scheme under the BIS Act, 1986. Standards covering more than 450 different food products have been published. Standards are laid for vegetable and fruit products, spices and condiments, animal products and processed foods. Once these standards are accepted, manufacturers whose products confirm to these standards are allowed to use BIS label on each unit of their product. The products are checked for quality by the BIS testing laboratories at Delhi, Mumbai, Calcutta, Chennai, Chandigarh and Patna. Some of the items which require compulsory BIS certification under PFA are natural food colours and food colour preparation, food additives, infant milk foods; milk cereal based weaning foods, milk powder and condensed milk.

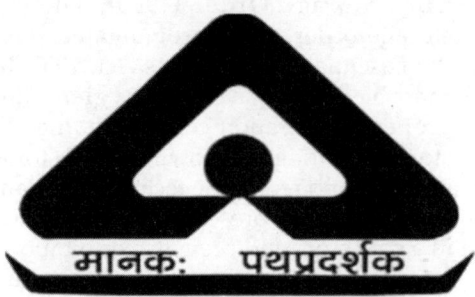

Bureau of Indian Standards

The AGMARK Standard

The word "AGMARK" is agricultural marketing. The AGMARK standard was set up by the directorate of marketing and inspection of the Government of India by introducing an Agricultural Produce Act in 1937. The word "AGMARK" seal ensures quality and purity. A sample AGMARK seal is given below:

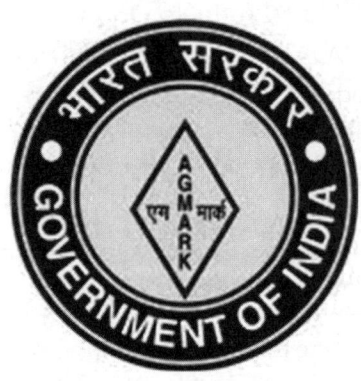

The Act defines quality of cereals, spices, oil seeds, oil, butter, ghee, legumes and eggs and provides for the categorization of commodities into various grades depending on the degree of purity in each case. The grades incorporated are grades 1, 2, 3 and 4 or special, good, fair and ordinary.

The central AGMARK laboratory at Nagpur continuously carries out research and development works in this field. The "certificate of authorization," is granted only to those in the trade having adequate experience and standing in the market.

Export (Quality Control and Inspection) Act, 1963

The export inspection council is responsible for the operation of this Act. Under the Act, a large number of exportable commodities have been notified for compulsory pre-shipment inspection. The quality control and inspection of various export products is administered through a network of more than fifty offices located around major production centers and ports of shipment. In addition, organizations may be recognized as agencies for inspection and/or quality control. Recently, the government has exempted agriculture and food products, fruit products and fish and fishery products from compulsory pre-shipment inspections; provided that the exporter has a firm letter from the overseas buyer stating that the overseas buyer does not require pre-shipment inspection from official Indian inspection agencies.

Codex Alimentarius

The Codex Alimentarius Commission is an inter-governmental body was established in 1963. It has over 170 member countries within the framework of the joint FAO/WHO food standards programme established by the Food and Agriculture Organization (FAO) of the United Nations and the World Health Organization (WHO). Codex alimentarious sets guidelines and standards to ensure 'fair trade practices' and consumer protection in relation to the global trade of food. Its primary purpose is "protecting the health of consumers and ensuring fair practices in the food trade." The commission also promotes coordination of all food standards work undertaken by International Governmental and Non-Governmental Organizations (INGOs).

Consumer Protection Act (1986)

The Act came into effect first on December 24, 1986 after being passed by the Indian parliament. It was modified later on and the modifications came into effect on March 15, 2003. The Act makes provisions to include both tangible goods and intangible service purchased from trader or service provider.

The main objective of this Act is to promote and protect the rights of the consumers, with regard to defective goods, deficiency of services, overcharging or any other unfair trade practices. Complaints can be referred to the district consumer redressal forum. The forum can order the opposite party for removal of the defect, replacement of the goods, return of the prices or charges or order payment of compensation for the loss or damage suffered due to deficiency of service. Appeals can be made to state commission and then to national commission.

Consumer Disputes Redressal Agencies

This section of the Act provides for the creation of consumer courts. The central government is given the responsibility to create and maintain the National Consumer Disputes Redressal Commission in New Delhi. The state government is given the responsibility to create a state consumer disputes redressal commission at the state level and a district consumer redressal forum at the district level. World consumer day is celebrated every year on 15th March.

STUDY QUESTIONS

1. What is adulteration? What problems arise due to adulteration?
2. What are the major types of adulteration?
3. What are the major food adulterants? How will you test the presence of these adulterants?
4. List the laws promulgated for the prevention of adulteration.
5. Write short notes on the following:
   a. Food Product Order
   b. AGMARK and BIS
   c. Codex Alimentarious
   d. Milk and Milk Products Order (1992)

9 Food Poisoning and Infection

Food is important for life and contains various life nourishing components. Though food is life nourishing but it could be toxic and can cause poisoning. Food poisoning may be due to poisons derived from plant and animal sources or due to chemicals added or preservatives at too high concentrations, or due to the presence of harmful microorganisms or toxins produced by them. The time from the consumption of poisonous food to the beginning of the symptoms varies from 10 minutes to 2 hours with same forms of chemicals, to around 6 hours with bacterial toxins, 12–72 hours when poisoning is due to living bacteria and 2–3 days, when poisonous mushrooms are the cause.

DEFINITION

Food poisoning is defined as the disorder of digestive system caused by eating certain foods, contaminated with certain microorganisms (that contain or produce toxins).

Food Poisoning by Microorganisms

Food Poisoning by Bacteria

The types of food involved in food poisoning are those favoring growth of causative organisms, so that a large number of bacteria or their products are present at the time of taking food. Food may be contaminated with bacteria at its source either in the animal as with meat, fish, milk or eggs obtained from infected animal, or from soil, as with vegetables or indirectly from contaminated water used in the preparation of food, by fly borne infections or by handling of food by man.

The bacteria that cause food poisoning are described as under:

1. **Staphylococcus aureus:** *Staphylococcus* is abbreviated to "*S. aureus*" or "*Staph aureus*" in medical literature. *S. aureus* was discovered in Aberdeen, Scotland in 1880 by the surgeon Sir Alexander Ogston in pus from surgical abscesses. *Staphylococcus* is salt tolerant and can grow in salty foods. As the germ multiplies in food, it produces toxins that can cause illness. Staphylococcal toxins are resistant to heat and cannot be destroyed by cooking. Foods at highest risk of contamination with *Staphylococcus aureus* and subsequent toxin production are those that are made by hand and require no cooking.

What does S. aureus cause?

In this bacterial poisoning cells or exotoxins produced are the cause of food poisioning. Since the exotoxins are absorbed by the gut wall they are also called enterotoxins. Enterotoxins are preferred in the food by the growth of the organisms and although the bacterial cells may be killed by heating and cooking, many of the enterotoxins are heat resistant and cause poisoning.

Transmission of Staphylococcus aureus

S. aureus is transmitted through air droplets or aerosol. When an infected person coughs or sneezes, numerous small droplets of saliva that remains suspended in air. These contain the bacteria and can infect others. It may also transmit through direct contact with objects that are contaminated by the bacteria or by bites from infected persons or animals.

Food products

Food products associated with this food poisoning are milk products such as curd, cream, custard, puddings, some pastries, sandwiches and sweets and prepared meat. Staphylococci multiply fast at ordinary temperature in the foods and release toxins. Pasteurized milk is also contaminated with staphylococci. The infection may also come from the udders of cow, buffalo or goat.

Symptoms of staphylococcal food poisoning

Staphylococcal toxins are fast acting, sometimes causing illness in as little as 30–45 minutes. Symptoms usually develop within one to six hours after eating contaminated food. Patients typically experience the following:

- Nausea
- Vomiting
- Stomach cramps
- Diarrhea

The illness is usually mild and most patients recover after one to three days. In a small minority of patients the illness may be more severe.

Diagnosis

Diagnosis of staphylococcal food poisoning in an individual is generally based only on the signs and symptoms of the patient. Presence of *S. aureus* in culture is normally insignificant since this bacterium is normally present on the skin, nose and pharynx of many humans and animals. The organism is readily cultured from nasopharynx or skin, or by culture of suspicious lesions.

Prevention of S. aureus food poisoning

The food poisoning can be prevented by:
- Washing hands and under fingernails vigorously with soap and water before handling and preparing food.
- Not preparing or serving food having wounds or skin infections.
- Keeping kitchens and food-serving areas clean and sanitized.
- Avoiding the preparation of food during nose or eye infection.

- Storing food at proper temperatures such as, keep hot foods hot (over 140 °F) and cold foods cold (40 °F or under).
- Storing cooked food in a wide, shallow container.
- By refrigerating the food as soon as possible.

2. **Clostridium botulinum (botulism)**: *Clostridium botulinum*, is a spore forming, anerobic microorganisms found in the soil. The spores are heat-resistant and can survive in foods that are incorrectly or minimally processed. The food poisoning caused by *Clostridium botulinum* is Botulism.

What does Clostridium botulinum cause?

The food containing *Clostridium botulinum* when ingested is absorbed through the mucosa of the stomach and upper part of the intestine and is so powerful that the fatal dose for a man may be as low as 0.01 mg. The toxin affects the nervous system by preventing the releasing of acetylcholine (neurotransmitter) at the presynaptic membrane of terminal knobs.

Transmission of Clostridium botulinum

Botulism is life-threatening bacterial illness. *Clostridium botulinum* bacteria grows on food and produces toxins that, when ingested, cause paralysis.

Food products

Improperly canned foods, baked potato, cooked meat, smoked or raw fish, cured pork and ham, honey or corn syrup, and home-canned vegetables. The foods such as oil infused with garlic and baked potatoes may also contain the bacteria.

Symptoms of botulism

Neurotoxins produced during botulism prevent neurotransmitters from functioning properly and motor control is inhibited. As botulism progresses, the patient experiences paralysis from top to bottom, starting with the eyes and face and moving to the throat, chest, and extremities.

Symptoms of botulism generally appear 12 to 72 hours after eating contaminated food. With treatment, illness lasts from 1 to 10 days.

In general, symptoms of botulism poisoning include the following:

- Nausea
- Vomiting
- Fatigue
- Dizziness
- Dry skin, mouth and throat
- Drooping eyelids
- Difficulty in swallowing
- Slurred speech
- Muscle weakness
- Body ache
- Paralysis
- Blurred vision
- Lack of fever

Full recovery from botulism poisoning can take weeks to months. Some people never fully recover.

Diagnosis

For diagnosing botulism, blood, stool or gastric secretion sample test will be done.

Prevention of botulism

The most important way of preventing botulism is maintaining the proper hygienic conditions in the kitchen and in the surroundings. Further, the canned food should not be taken if they smells bad or bulge. The food should be thoroughly cleaned and left over food should be kept in the refrigerator. The potatoes should not be stored at room temperature. The foods should not be left, if they are cooked at home at temperatures between 40 and 140 °F (4.5 to 60 °C) for more than four hours.

Food Poisoning by Moulds

Aspergillus flavus

Aspergillus flavus is a plant, animal and human pathogen that produces the carcinogen, aflatoxin. Aspergillus flavus is a fungus. It grows by producing thread like branching filaments known as hyphae. Filamentous fungi such as A. flavus are sometimes also called molds.

What does A. flavus cause?

The bacteria secrete the toxin called aflatoxin which is carcinogenic. Aspergillus flavus is also the second leading cause of aspergillosis (fungal growth in lungs) in humans.

Transmission of Aspergillus flavus

Aspergillus is a fungus whose spores are present in the air we breathe, but does not normally cause illness. However, an individual with a weakened immune status may be susceptible to aspergillus infection. Since the spores of the fungus are present in air and through soil it can be spread.

Food products

Aflatoxins grow on grains and legumes mostly during storage, so the grains and legumes must be stored correctly to limit this problem. The foods such as peanuts, whole grains, nuts and fish contain aflatoxins.

Symptoms of A. flavus poisoning

The symptoms of A. flavus poisoning includes:

- Fever
- Wheezing
- Shortness of breath
- Unintentional weight loss
- Fatigue
- Fever and chills
- Cough that brings up blood-streaked sputum (hemoptysis)
- Chest or joint pain
- Nosebleed
- Facial swelling on one side
- Skin lesions

Diagnosis and prevention

For diagnosing A. flavus poisoning blood test have to be done. Prevention includes the proper storage, handling and maintaining the hygienic conditions in the surroundings.

Foodborne Infection

A foodborne infection is caused by the ingestion of food containing pathogenic microorganisms (i.e. bacteria, virus or parasite) which multiply in the gastrointestinal tract and produces widespread inflammation.

The most commonly implicated microorganisms include species of Salmonella, Shigella, E. coli, etc.

The foodborne infections by certain bacteria are described as under:

1. **Salmonella:** *Salmonella* is a genus of rodshaped, gram-negative, non-spore-forming, predominantly motile entero-bacteria. There are various species of *Salmonellae* which vary in their degree of effectiveness. *Salmonella typhimurium* and *Salmonella enteritidis* are the most common types which cause infection in the individual. The infection caused by *Salmonella* is known as salmonellosis.

What does Salmonella cause?
Salmonella establishes in the alimentary canal of the host. In a week the bacterial cell disintegrates and releases poisonous substances called endotoxin which affects the individual cause salmonellosis.

Transmission of salmonellosis
Salmonellosis usually spread by eating food contaminated with *salmonella* or due to poor handling of food. *Salmonella* may also spread through the feces of some pets, especially those with diarrhea.

Food products
Beef, poultry, milk and eggs are most often infected with *Salmonella*. But vegetables may also be contaminated. Contaminated foods usually look and smell normal.

Symptoms of salmonellosis
- Diarrhea
- Fever
- Abdominal cramps
- Headache
- Nausea
- Vomiting
- Loss of appetite

The symptoms appear 12 to 72 hours after infection, and the illness usually lasts 4 to 7 days.

Diagnosis
Salmonellosis is diagnosed based on a medical history and a physical examination will be done. A stool culture and blood tests will also be done to diagnose salmonellosis.

Prevention
Salmonellosis can be best prevented as:
- By not eating raw or undercooked eggs, as these are used for making several dishes.
- Food should be cooked well and should be handled with proper sanitation and hygiene.
- Avoid raw or unpasteurized milk or other dairy products.
- Fruits and vegetables should be washed before consumption.
- Uncooked meats should be kept separately.
- Hands should be washed before handling and cooking of food.
- The patients suffering with salmonellosis should be kept away from kitchen and they should not be allowed to touch the utensils and other items meant for food preparation.

Diet in salmonellosis
To prevent dehydration, take frequent sips of a rehydration drink. It is advisable to stay on your normal diet as this will help in providing adequate nutrition but it is also recommended that foods such as spicy foods, alcohol and coffee are avoided till the full recovery.

2. **Shigella:** *Shigella* is a kind of bacteria that is a most common cause of diarrhea in humans. They are microscopic living creatures that pass from person to person. *Shigella* was discovered over 100 years ago by a Japanese scientist named Shiga, for whom they are named. There are several different kinds of *Shigella* bacteria: *Shigella sonnei*, also known as "Group D" *Shigella*, accounts for over two-thirds of shigellosis. Shigellosis is an infectious disease caused by a group of bacteria called *Shigella*.

What does Shigella cause?
Shigella produces strains called enterotoxin and shigatoxin which causes are associated with causing hemolytic anemia, acute kidney failure, and low platelet count.

Transmission of Shigella
The *shigella* bacteria pass from one infected person to the next. *Shigella* infections may be acquired from eating contaminated food. Flies which breed in infected feces and then

contaminate food can transmit *Shigella*. Water may become contaminated with *Shigella* bacteria, if sewage runs into it.

Food products
It usually develops as a result of drinking contaminated water although it can be contracted by eating foods which have been in contact with infected water. One example of this is salads which are often washed in water before use.

Symptoms
- Nausea
- Stomach cramps
- Vomiting
- Severe diarrhea which often contains blood and mucus
- Fever
- Rectal spasms

The incubation period —the time from the initial consumption to the appearance of these symptoms is usually 1 to 2 days. However, these symptoms can appear after as little as 12 hours.

Diagnosis
For detecting the shigellosis, stool test will be done.

Prevention: Shigellosis can be prevented by:
- Maintaining proper hygienic conditions in the surroundings and in the cooking area.
- By washing hands with soap carefully and frequently, especially after going to the bathroom, after changing diapers, and before preparing foods or beverages.
- By disposing of spoiled diapers properly.
- By keeping the infected children with diarrhea out of child care settings.
- By supervising handwashing of toddlers and small children after they use the toilet.
- By not preparing food for others when suffering with infection.
- By not using the water of the places which are dirty and contaminated.

3. **Escherichia coli (E. coli):** Commonly abbreviated *E. coli* is a gram-negative, rod-shaped bacterium that is commonly found in the small intestine of warm blooded organisms (endotherms). Most *E. coli* strains are harmless, but some can cause serious food infection to the human, and are also responsible for food contamination. The food infection caused by *E. coli* leads to bloody diarrhea, anemia and kidney failure, which sometimes leads to death.

What does E. coli cause?
E. coli lives inside intestines, where it helps in breaking down of food and digestion of the food. But sometimes, certain types of strains of *E. coli* can get from the intestines into the blood, which causes infection.

Transmission of E. coli
E. coli infection is transmitted by coming in contact with the feces, or stool of humans or animals. *E. coli* is also transmitted by drinking water or eating food that has been contaminated by *E. coli.*

Food products
The food products in which *E. coli* can develop are meat which are not well cooked, raw milk or dairy products. Bacteria can also spread from a cow's udders to its milk, raw fruits and vegetables are also the foods which when consumed without washing and cutting can spread *E. coli* infection.

E. coli in water
The water of lakes, pools and water supplies, is also an important cause of *E. coli* infection.

The bacteria can also spread from one person to another, usually when an infected person does not wash his or her hands well after a bowel movement. *E. coli* can spread from an infected person's hands to other people or to objects.

What are the symptoms?
The main symptoms of an *E. coli* infection are:
- Bloody diarrhea
- Vomiting
- Nausea
- Pale skin
- Fever
- Weakness
- Passing only small amounts of urine

Symptoms usually start 3 or 4 days after you come in contact with the *E. coli*.

Children are more likely than adults to have symptoms. Many patients get better in about a week.

Diagnosis
E. coli infection will be diagnosed by stool culture test.

Prevention
Food and water that are infected with *E. coli* germs look and smell normal. But there are some things you can do to prevent infection:
- All types of meat should be cooked at temperature of 160 °F (71 °C).
- The hands should be washed with soap before start working in the kitchen, especially after touching raw meat.
- The kitchen utensils should be washed thoroughly.
- Only pasteurized milk should be used.
- The drinking water should be chlorinated at a regular interval of time and if filter is used it should be serviced and cleaned.
- The hands should be washed with soap after using toilets and after changing diapers.
- The hygiene in the surroundings should be maintained.

4. **Bacillus cereus:** *B. cereus* is a rod-shaped gram-positive bacteria which produces strains and causes food poisoning.

What does B. cereus cause?
Bacillus cereus or *B. cereus* is a type of bacteria that produces toxins. These toxins can cause two types of illness:

Type I: Characterized by diarrhea

Type II: Called emetic toxin, characterized by nausea and vomiting.

These bacteria are present in foods and can multiply quickly at room temperature.

Transmission of Bacillus cereus
Bacillus cereus is widespread in the environment and enters the food chain through contaminated food and water.

Food products
A variety of foods, particularly rice and leftovers, as well as sauces, soups, and other prepared foods that have set out too long at room temperature.

What are the symptoms?
The main symptoms of this infection are:
- Watery diarrhea
- Vomiting
- Nausea
- Abdominal cramps

The symptoms may develop within:

Diarrheal: 6–15 hours

Emetic (vomiting): 30 minutes to 6 hours

Diagnosis
Diagnosis depends on the *B. cereus* poisoning symptoms.

Prevention
- Food should not be stored longer than two hours, keep hot foods hot (over 140 °F) and cold foods cold (40 °F or under).
- Cooked food should be stored in a shallow container and refrigerator.

STUDY QUESTIONS

1. What is food poisoning? What are its causes?
2. What are the effects of food poisoning caused by *Staphylococcus aureus*?
3. What is Salmonellosis?
4. Give short notes on:
   a. *Clostridium botulinum*
   b. Symptoms of food poisoning
   c. Prevention of botulism
   d. Diagnosis of *S. aureus* poisoning

10 Science of Food Preparation

Preparing the food is an art. As before drawing we think about the technique that helps in giving the structures more beautiful looks similarly before preparation of our food we think about the techniques that will help in making the food tastier and acceptable. Like in art the items are collected before drawing, in the same way before food preparation, food preparing items are collected according to the need and type of food which have to cook.

Food preparation is not an easy task. Preparation of food generally requires the selection, addition and combining of ingredients in an appropriate manner, so that food cooked tastes good and becomes acceptable by everyone and also food becomes nutritionally adequate for everyone. But all these factors depend on the techniques involved in preparing the food.

WHY THE FOOD IS COOKED?

1. The flavor of the foods is improved during cooking. The use of spices and condiments adds taste and flavor.
2. The physical and chemical changes in the food whereby colour, texture and appearance may be improved and palatability, acceptability and the digestibility of the food is also increased.
3. The same food cooked in different ways provides variety in the diet. For example, the carrots can be eaten in raw form, in salad form and also added during vegetable preparation.
4. The digestibilities of foods are also increased as during cooking the food softens.

5. Cooking enchances the availability of some nutrients. For example, trypsin inhibitor present in protein foods is destroyed by cooking. This makes the trypsin freely available to the body. Similarly, starch is more easily available to the body after cooking.
6. The bacteria and other microorganisms are killed during cooking of food and the keeping quality of foods also improves.

Techniques of Food Preparation

Different, traditional and modern methods of cooking are discussed below:

A. *Dry heat*: By this method following techniques are involved:

Broiling or grilling

This is the most ancient and simplest method of cooking. In this, the food is exposed directly to heat either of a gas flame, electric wires or coals. The important condition is that the heat should be strong enough so that the food is thoroughly cooked. In broiling or grilling, the fire should be free from smoke, or ash, otherwise the food will become sooty. A little salt sprinkled on the fire will keep it clean.

For pan broiling, a hot metal pan or top of the stove is used. But the pan should be greased by enough fat so that the food will not stick to the pot.

Merits

1. Enhances flavor, appearance and taste of the product.
2. It requires less time to cook.
3. Minimum fat is used.

Demerits

1. Constant attention is required to prevent charring.
2. A loss of nutrients also occurs.

Baking

Baking is done in an electric 'oven.' In oven, enclosed air is heated and food is cooked. For good cooking it is necessary that the food should be properly placed in the oven and the temperature should also be evenly distributed throughout. Biscuits, bread, cakes, vegetable pies and puddings are baked.

Merits

1. Baking lends a unique baked flavor to foods.
2. Foods become light and fluffy — cakes, custards, bread.
3. Certain foods can be prepared only by this method — bread, cakes.
4. Uniform and bulk cooking can be achieved, e.g. bun, bread.
5. Flavor and texture are improved.
6. Variety of dishes can be made.

Demerits

1. Special equipment like oven is required.
2. Baking skills are necessary to obtain a product with ideal, texture, flavor and colour.
3. Careful monitoring needed to prevent scorching.

Earthen oven (tandoor)

A tandoor is a little ordinary oven. It is the cheapest medium of cooking food. A tandoor is a hollow, round in shape. Before using it is heated up with the fire. After heating the chapattis or nans are made and pasted on the inside walls of the oven. The food items such as seekh kababs, tandoori fish and chicken are cooked in a tandoor.

Merits

The food cooked have a delicious taste.

Demerits

It is a time taking method of cooking.

Roasting

Roasting is to cook food over an open fire. The food is cooked thoroughly so that all surfaces of food are equally heated. Roasting is also done by putting sand in a deep frying pan. The food items such as grams, peanuts, sweet potatoes and puffed rice are roasted. The sand is put, in a deep frying pan *(karahi)* and when it becomes hot, the peanut or gram or corn will be put in it. Sometimes roasting is done by using a little fat as medium, such as groundnuts are roasted by pouring oil or other fat. In this method very little fat is used, from time to time. Roasting is a quick method of cooking but some of the vitamin contents of food are destroyed as food cooked comes directly in touch with fire.

Merits

1. Quick method of cooking.
2. It improves the appearance, flavor and texture of the food.
3. Spices are easily powdered, if they are first roasted.

Demerits

1. Food can be scorched due to carelessness.
2. Roasting denatures proteins reducing their availability.

B. *Moist heat*: Cooking by moist heat includes boiling, stewing, braising and steaming.

Boiling

Boiling is the most common method of cooking food. In boiling, the food items are completely immersed in water and boils at 100 °C. The food items such as root vegetables, cereals, pulses and meat because of their toughness require cooking through boiling. If the food is boiled continuously, water is evaporated quickly and the water and texture of the food also change continuously. Mostly, vegetables are simmered in a small amount of water.

Merits

1. It is an easy method of cooking and does not require constant attention.
2. Foods cooked by this method are soft and are recommended for patients during illness.

Demerits

1. The big disadvantage of this method is that it wastes fuel.

2. It breaks the food and spoils its appearance.
3. There also occurs the loss of heat labile nutrients. Some valuable nutrients and flavors are lost when the cooking water is discarded.

Stewing

In stewing, the cooking is carried out in a small quantity of water. The food will be kept, in a covered pan, over mild heat, below the boiling point of water for a long period. The cooking utensil is tightly covered to avoid evaporation. Food to be stewed should be cut in small pieces to get it cooked well. The use of water should be limited and lastly the heat provided should be slow and steady to avoid over cooking. Stewing is suitable for cooking tough foods such as meat, pulses and dried vegetables to make them tender and digestible. Since foodstuffs are cooked in covered pans and the juices are retained as gravy, stewed foods are nourishing.

Merits

1. It does not need constant and frequent attention.
2. Flavor is retained.

Demerits

1. Some of the valuable contents of the food, chiefly vitamin C, are destroyed because of the slow process of cooking.
2. The process is time consuming and there is wastage of fuel.

Blanching

Some foods have the outer coverings which are needed to be peeled off without making them tender. This can be achieved by blanching. In this method, food is dipped in boiling water for 5 seconds to 2 minutes depending on the texture of the food. This helps to remove the skin or peel without softening the food. Blanching can also be done by pouring enough boiling water on the food to immerse it for some time or subjecting foods to boiling temperatures for short periods and then immediately immersing in cold water. The process causes the skin to become loose and can be peeled off easily.

Merits

1. Peels can be easily removed to improve digestibility.
2. Destroys enzymes that bring about spoilage.
3. Texture can be maintained while improving the colour and flavor of food.

Demerits

1. Loss of nutrients, if cooking water is discarded.

Braising

Braising is the most common method used in everyday life. Braising is a combined method of roasting and stewing in a pan with a tight fitting lid. Flavorings and seasonings are added and food is allowed to cook gently. The vegetable and meat is first made slightly brown in hot fat and then cooked in little water. By doing so there is no loss of nutrients as moisture is entirely used up.

Steaming

In steaming the food does not come into direct contact with water. Steaming is done by two ways:

Direct method: In this, the steam is applied directly to the food which is placed in a perforated rack over boiling water in a pan which is tightly covered with a lid. For example— idlis.

Indirect method: The food is packed into a vessel with a lid. The vessel is then immersed in another vessel of boiling water (double boiler). The heat for cooking the food is supplied by the boiling water all round the immersed inner vessel, as in the making of puddings.

Merits

1. Less chance of burning and scorching.
2. Texture of food is better as it becomes light and fluffy.
3. Cooking time is less and fuel wastage is less.
4. Steamed foods like idli and idiappam contain less fat and are easily digested and are good for children, aged and for therapeutic diets.
5. Nutrient loss is minimised.

Demerits
1. Steaming equipment is required.
2. This method is limited to the preparation of selected foods.

Cooking under pressure
In this the steam under pressure is used and the device used is pressure cooker. In pressure cooking, food is placed in a sealed container with very little water and cooked by the pressure of steam. As the temperature is elevated quickly in the food cooked with steam under pressure, the cooking period is reduced and also the loss of heat-labile nutrients occur. It is a useful device nowadays as it saves fuel and time. The food can be cooked rapidly. Different dishes of the meal can be prepared at a time. There is a loss of vitamin C and other soluble vitamins and minerals.

The cooker should not be filled more than 2/3 of its capacity. The lid used should be air-tight. The 'weight' should be put on when there is complete pressure inside and it starts making a hissing sound. The time should be checked properly and after the food is cooked, it should be cooled slowly. The pressure cooker and its various components should be thoroughly cleaned after use.

Merits
1. Cooking time is less compared to other methods.
2. Nutrient and flavor loss is minimised.
3. Conserves fuel and time as different items can be cooked at the same time.
4. Less chance for burning and scorching.
5. Constant attention is not necessary.

Demerits
1. The initial investment may not be affordable to everybody.
2. Knowledge of the usage, care and maintenance of cooker is required to prevent accidents.
3. Careful watch on the cooking time is required to prevent overcooking.

C. *Frying*: Frying is a quick method of cooking because of the high temperature that is used. Fat is used for frying the food.

Fat has a very much higher boiling point than water. It needs continuous careful attention. Frying can be done by different ways:

i. **Sauteing:** A small quantity of fat is used, which is just sufficient to be absorbed by the food cooked in it. The food is turned frequently.

ii. **Shallow frying:** The food is cooked in a lightly greased pan. Sufficient quantity of fat is used in the pan and food is turned to cook both sides equally. Food items such as— paratha, omlette, pancake and tikki are shallow fried. The fat should be drained by using absorbent paper before serving.

iii. **Deep frying:** The food is immersed in a deep pan or kadahi containing excess quantity of fat or oil. Potato chips, bonda, pakoras and puris are deep fat fried.

For satisfactory results, food should be fried in fats and oils heated to 320 °C. At this temperature a faint blue fume or smoke rises from the fat or oil. If the food is introduced into the hot fat or oil before the blue fume rises, then the fat will penetrate into the food and make it sodden, soggy and greasy. The fat should not be overheated, as overheating causes browning and burning of the foods outside, while the interior may remain uncooked.

Merits
1. Very quick method of cooking.
2. The calorific values of foods are increased since fat is used as the cooking media.
3. Frying lends a delicious flavor and attractive appearance to foods.
4. Taste and texture are improved.

Demerits
1. Careful monitoring is required as food easily gets charred when the smoking temperature is not properly maintained.
2. The food may become soggy due to too much oil absorption.
3. Fried foods are not easily digested.

4. Repeated use of heated oils will have ill effects on health.

5. Losses of vitamins occur.

D. *Solar cooking*: The food is cooked in a device known as solar cooker. It is a method of cooking food by converting the solar energy into heat energy. A solar cooker is placed at such an angle that the mirror reflects the sun's rays into the food placed in the container. The containers are blackened to absorb the maximum of the sun's heat. This is an economical method of cooking as it saves fuel and electricity. But the disadvantage is that it takes time to cook food.

E. *Infrared radiation or microwave cookery*: This is the advanced method of cooking. The food to be cooked is placed in an electronic oven where it is exposed to the penetration of microwaves produced by a magnetron tube. The microwaves cause agitation of the molecules within the food so that heat is generated. Cooking time is shortened to ten times less than may be needed by conventional methods.

The flavor and nutritive values of vegetables are good in comparison with other methods of cooking.

The disadvantages of microwave cookery are that food is only cooked in small quantities and the food is unattractive to look at, as it does not brown the food. Time has to be adjusted carefully to avoid over-cooking. The equipment is still too expensive for household use.

Changes in Food during Preparation

However, nutritious a meal is, it needs to be attractive in appearance and flavor, if it is to be eaten and the nutrients made use of. It must stimulate the appetite. The art of food preparation is the art of skilful combination of colour, texture and flavor to please the eyes, the nose and the palate.

Changes in Colour

Food undergoes many colour changes during cooking, some of which enhance the desirability of the product, whereas others do not. Fruits and vegetables have attractive colours but during cooking, the colour is changed due to the pH of the cooking medium.

Effect of Heat

The change in the plant pigment called chlorophyll, is affected due to heat. The green colour of the leafy vegetables is changed to olive green and then to brown in the long run, especially when an acid medium is used. Carotenoids, the red pigments, present in peaches and carrots, leach out into the cooking medium making the food look pale in appearance. The colour of meat is due to a red pigment in muscle called myoglobin and also due to blood pigment called hemoglobin. The red colour of meat is changed to pink, grey or brown upon exposure to heat.

Effect of Alkali

In food baking, soda (alkali) is used to maintain the green colour, but it destroys the vitamin C and thiamine content of the food. It is advisable to maintain the good colour by cooking the green leafy vegetables in an uncovered utensil or leaving the pan uncovered for the first few minutes of cooking.

The pale yellow colour of onions, asparagus and apple is due to flavonoid pigments. Alkaline tap water is liable to cause them to turn into a deep yellow-brown colour on cooking which can be prevented by adding an acid such as a little lemon juice. Yellowing of rice can also be prevented in this way.

Changes in Texture

Texture is the physical state of the food. The intake of food very much depends on the texture of food. Raw foods undergo many changes during preparation of food.

On heating, the proteins coagulate. For example, egg white coagulates and becomes solid when heated. When milk is heated, a scum is formed on cooling; this is due to the protein coagulation. The addition of citric acid in hot milk coagulates it very fast by separating casein, the protein part of milk.

Coagulation is better at low temperature. Overheating makes the substance stringy and tough.

However, some proteins do not coagulate on heating. Collagen and elastin, the two important insoluble proteins in meat, become tough on cooking by heat; so in order to make the connective tissues of meat tender, the meat should be cooked by moist heat.

The texture of cereals, fruits and vegetables is related to the cellulose fibres. The cellulose becomes soft on cooking but loses its shape on overcooking. In case of cereals, cooking gelatinizes the starch, softens and breaks down the cellulose framework of the plant. When starch is cooked by using dry heat, it darkens in colour as the starch is converted into dextrins which are more easily digested than starch.

Flavor

Cooking also improves and brings flavors in food. Flavor is sensed by taste and smell. Good flavored food encourages formation of saliva in the mouth which is helpful in digesting food. The physical and chemical changes bring changes in flavors which are brought about during cooking processes. The addition of spices and essences are used in cooking to improve the flavor. Highly flavored foods should be wrapped in aluminium foil to retain the maximum inherent flavor, which is lost when it is cooked unwrapped.

MINIMIZING NUTRIENT WATER INPUT AND OUTPUT

1. Choose fresh foods that are not over-ripe, bruised, cut or scraped.
2. Foods should be stored in a dark place.
3. Always cook the whole food or if the peel is unpalatable remove it.
4. Use less quantity of water for steaming the food.
5. The food should not be cooked for a longer period of time.
6. The food once cooked should be eaten immediately, otherwise microorganisms may develop.
7. Use of baking soda should be avoided as this increases loss of vitamin C.
8. Always cut the large pieces of raw food.
9. Copper utensils should not be used for food preparation as the copper destroys vitamin C.

STUDY QUESTIONS

1. What are the reasons of cooking food?
2. What are the methods of cooking food by using dry heat?
3. What are the changes that occur in the texture and flavor during food preparation?
4. Write short notes on:
   a. Steaming
   b. Shallow frying
5. How the nutrient water input and output is minimized?

11 Malnutrition

Malnutrition is the one of the biggest problems of India. Besides remarkable achievements and overall economic growth of 8% over the last five years, a major portion of India's population is undernourished. According to the current statistics of India, 2012, 48% children under the age of five are stunted (too short for their age), which indicates that half of the country's children are chronically malnourished.

Malnutrition is globally the most important risk factor for illness and death. The consequences of child undernutrition for morbidity and mortality are enormous and there is, in addition, an appreciable impact of undernutrition on productivity so that a failure to invest in combating nutrition reduces potential economic growth. Moreover, inequalities in undernutrition between demographic, socioeconomic and geographic groups increased during the 1990s.

The worst performing states in India with underweight children under five years of age are Madhya Pradesh (60 percent), Jharkhand (56.5 percent) and Bihar (55.9 percent). Similarly anemia prevalence among children (6–59 months) is more than 70 percent in Bihar, Madhya Pradesh, Uttar Pradesh, Haryana, Chhattisgarh, Andhra Pradesh, Karnataka and Jharkhand.

What is Malnutrition?

Malnutrition is a broad term which refers to both **undernutrition** (subnutrition) and **overnutrition**. Malnutrition occurs when the diet of the individual does not provide adequate calories and protein for maintenance and growth. Malnutrition also occurs due to consumption of too many calories, this condition will be called overnutrition.

According to WHO: Malnutrition is defined as *the cellular imbalance between supply of nutrients and energy and the body's demand for them to ensure growth, maintenance and specific functions.* Malnutrition can also be defined as the *insufficient, excessive or imbalanced consumption of nutrients. Several different nutritional disorders may develop, depending on which nutrients are lacking or consumed in excess.*

ECOLOGY OF MALNUTRITION

Malnutrition occurs due to the lack of essential nutrients, resulting in poorer health, may be caused by a number of conditions or circumstances. Malnutrition is usually caused by:

- **Food shortages:** Due to increase in population food shortage is also occurring. The families having more number of people are unable to feed their family. Secondly due to lack of technology needed for higher yields found in modern agriculture, such as nitrogen fertilizers, pesticides and irrigation. Food shortages are a significant cause of malnutrition in many parts of the world.

- **Digestive disorders and stomach conditions:** People having malabsorption problems suffer from malnutrition as their bodies cannot absorb the nutrients they need for good health. Examples include patients with ulcerative colitis. Such patients have lack of essential nutrients in the body and thus suffer from malnutrition. The children suffering from diarrhea, intestinal parasites and gastrointestinal disturbances suffer from malnutrition.

- **Mental health problems:** People with mental problems have conditions, such as depression, may skip their meals which lead to malnutrition.
- **Drinking:** The people who drinks lot suffers from alcoholism, as the body becomes dependent on alcohol and they do not eat their meals and thus malnutrition occurs. Individuals who suffer from alcoholism can develop gastritis, or pancreas damage. These problems also seriously hamper the body's ability to digest food, absorb certain vitamins, and produce hormones which regulate metabolism. Alcohol contains calories, reducing the patient's feeling of hunger, so he/she consequently, may not eat enough proper food to supply the body with essential nutrients.
- **Poverty:** Poverty is the true determinant of malnutrition in society. The children belonging to the poor family always have a scarcity of food. Due to poor or inadequate diet, the lack of nutrients in the body occurs which ultimately leads to malnutrition. The people living in poor slums have inadequate sanitary environment which affects their quality of life and malnutrition occurs.
- **Lack of breastfeeding:** Women in the modern world do not feel necessary to breastfed their child which leads to malnutrition in infants and children. Another reason for lack of breastfeeding is that mothers do not know how to get their baby to latch on properly, or suffer pain and discomfort. In some parts of the world mothers due to illiteracy or lack of knowledge about the benefits of breastfeeding still believe that bottle feeding is better for the child.

PROTEIN ENERGY MALNUTRITION

Protein energy malnutrition (PEM) is one of the most important public health problems in many developing countries including India, South East Asia and Africa. Protein energy malnutrition refers to the condition which occurs due to the deficiency of protein and calories in the diet. PEM can occur in patients who have been hospitalized due to pain, loss of appetite, nausea and problems is swallowing, chewing, or digesting food. Diarrhea, bleeding, burns, trauma, infection, fever, certain medications, benign or malignant tumors, malabsorption disorders, kidney disease, and abnormally high blood glucose levels (glycosuria) can hasten the loss of nutrients. PEM can also occur in anorexic or bulimic individuals.

Classification of Protein Energy Malnutrition

PEM is identified by the children requiring nutritional or health interventions. Some of the classifications are given below:

Gomez Classification

The classification is based upon the weight retardation. The child's weight is compared to that of a normal child (50th percentile) of the same age. It is useful for population screening and public health evaluations.

Percent of reference weight for age= [(patient weight)/(weight of normal child of same age)] × 100

Classification	Definition	Grading	
Gomez	Weight below % median WFA	Mild (grade 1)	75–90% WFA
		Moderate (grade 2)	60–74% WFA
		Severe (grade 3)	< 60% WFA

Waterlow classification

Chronic malnutrition results in stunting. Malnutrition also affects the child's body proportions eventually resulting in body wastage. According to this classification:

- Percent weight for height = [(weight of patient)/(weight of a normal child of the same height)] × 100
- Percent height for age = [(height of patient)/(height of a normal child of the same age)] × 100

Table 11.1: Classification of malnutrition in children

	Mild malnutrition	Moderate malnutrition	Severe malnutrition
Percent ideal body weight	80–90%	70–79%	< 70%
Percent of usual body weight	90–95%	80–89%	< 80%
Albumin (g/dL)	2.8–3.4	2.1–2.7	< 2.1
Transferrin (mg/dL)	150–200	100–149	< 100
Total lymphocyte count (per µL)	1200–2000	800–1199	< 800

Types of Protein Energy Malnutrition (PEM)

There are four types of PEM:
- i. Primary PEM
- ii. Secondary PEM
- iii. Kwashiorkar
- iv. Marasmus

i. Primary PEM: When the diet does not provide adequate protein, the condition occurs is primary PEM.

ii. Secondary PEM: This is most common in the United States and is related to cancer, kidney failure, AIDS, inflammatory bowel disease, and illnesses reducing absorption and use of nutrients; depending on the patient's health, the organ may be negatively affected.

iii. Kwashiorkor: Kwashiorkor is also known as malignant malnutrition. Kwashiorkor is a form of malnutrition that occurs when there is not enough protein in the diet.

Kwashiorkor typically starts after the child has been weaned and breast milk has been replaced with a diet in low protein, although, it can occur in infants, if the mother is protein-deprived. Kwashiorkor can also occur due to parasites and infections that can interfere with nutritional status.

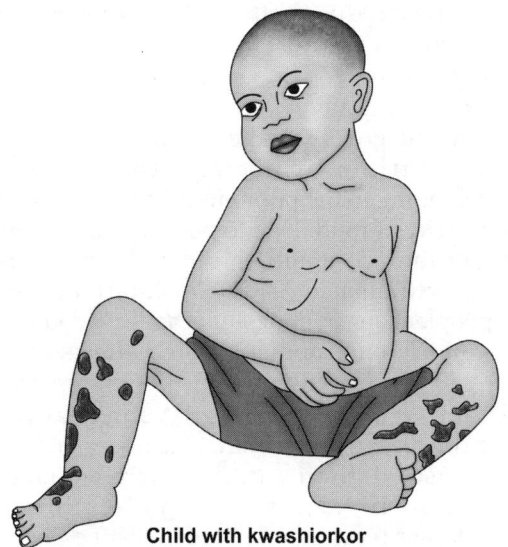
Child with kwashiorkor

Causes and risk factors
Kwashiorkor is most common in areas where there is:
- Famine
- Low protein diets
- Limited food supply
- Milk allergies in infants
- Fat diets
- Low levels of education (when people do not understand how to eat a proper diet)

Symptoms
- Hair changes (change in color or texture)
- Increased and more severe infections due to damaged immune system
- Irritability
- Large belly that sticks out (protrudes)
- Lethargy or apathy
- Changes in pigment of the skin
- Decreased muscle mass
- Diarrhea
- Shock (late stage)
- Swelling (edema)
- Failure to gain weight and growth
- Fatigue
- Loss of muscle mass
- Rash (dermatitis)

Signs
- An enlarged liver (hepatomegaly) and
- General swelling.

Tests: The following tests are done for diagnosing kwashiorkor:

1. **Arterial blood gas:** A blood gas is done to measure the level of oxygen and carbon dioxide in the blood. It also determines the acidity (pH) of blood. The test is used to evaluate respiratory diseases and conditions that affect the lungs. It helps to determine the effectiveness of oxygen therapy. The test also provides information about the body's acid–base balance, which can reveal important clues about lung and kidney function and the body's general metabolic state.

2. **BUN:** BUN stands for blood urea nitrogen. The test is performed to measure the amount of urea nitrogen in the blood formed by the destruction of proteins.

3. **Complete blood count:** A complete blood count (CBC) test is done to detect the problems related with RBC production and destruction. It also helps in diagnosing infection, allergies, and problems with blood clotting.

4. **Serum creatinine:** Creatinine is a breakdown product of creatine, which is an important part of muscle. The test is done to evaluate kidney function. Creatinine is removed from the body entirely by the kidneys. If kidney function is abnormal, creatinine levels will increase in the blood (because less creatinine is released through urine).

5. **Creatinine clearance:** The creatinine clearance test compares the level of creatinine in urine with the creatinine level in the blood. The test helps provide information on kidney function.

6. **Serum potassium:** This test measures the amount of potassium in the blood. This test is often done to diagnose nutritional problems, kidney disease or liver disease.

7. **Urinalysis:** Urinalysis is the physical, chemical, and microscopic examination of urine. It involves a number of tests to detect and measure various compounds that pass through the urine.

Treatment: The disease can be treated by incorporating calories and proteins in the diet. For treating kwashiorkor, the diet should have enough carbohydrates, fat (at least 10 percent of total calories), and protein (12 percent of total calories).

iv. **Marasmus:** Marasmus is one of the most serious forms of protein–energy malnutrition (PEM) in the world. It occurs when the diet lacks both protein and energy, the condition occurs is marasmus. This lack of nutrition can range from a shortage of certain vitamins to complete starvation.

Marasmus occurs most often in developing nations or in countries where poverty, along with inadequate food supplies and contaminated water, are prevalent. Marasmus often affects children in regions with high rates of poverty.

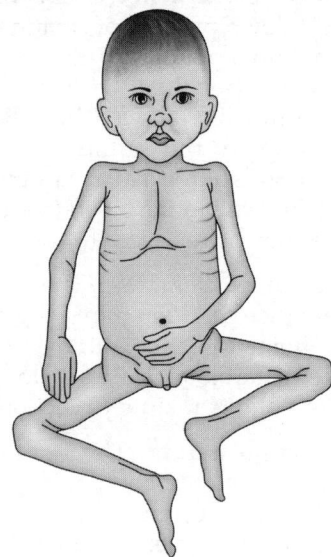

Child with marasmus

Causes and risk factors
- Contaminated water supplies
- Chronic hunger
- Poor, unbalanced diet lacking in grains, fruits and vegetables, and protein
- Inadequate food supplies
- Other vitamin deficiencies (vitamins A, E or K)

Symptoms

The symptoms of marasmus can range from mild to severe depending on the degree of malnutrition. The symptoms may also include:
- Chronic or persistent diarrhea
- Dizziness
- Unexplained weight loss
- Fatigue
- Change in level of consciousness or lethargy
- Full or partial paralysis of the legs
- Loss of bladder or bowel control
- Prolonged vomiting or diarrhea

Signs
- Retardation which is much more marked than that of length.
- Wasting of muscles
- Swelling of legs and feet
- Loose and wrinkled skin

- Abdomen protuberant
- Monkey face
- Increased appetite
- Patient is calm and quiet but crying all the time.
- Eyes are sunken and depressed
- Body temperature is subnormal.
- Infection is common.

Tests: The following test are done for diagnosing marasmus:
1. **Blood glucose analysis:** The test is done for detecting the blood glucose level in the body. If the level of blood glucose is <3 mmol/L, it may indicate the presence of hypoglycemia.
2. **Microscopy:** The test is done for detecting the presence of infection. The test involves examination of blood smears to check for presence of parasites. If tests are positive, doctors can confirm an infection.
3. **Urine examination and culture:** An infection can be indicated if there are over 10 leukocytes per high-power field.
4. **Albumin test:** If albumin level is found to be less than 35 g/L, it can indicate massive impairment of protein synthesis. This is not useful as a diagnostic test and is, rather helpful for prognosis.

Treatment

Treatment of marasmus involves a special feeding and rehydration plan and close medical observation to prevent and manage complications of malnutrition.

A nutritious, well-balanced diet containing adequate calories, high protein, carbohydrates, minerals and vitamins should be given to the patient. The diet must include food items such as fresh fruits and vegetables, grains and pulses. Nutrition education of mothers is also a necessary part of treatment. The mothers should be told to continue breastfeeding for as long as possible as this helps in improving the nutritional status of the child.

Marasmic Kwashiorkor

The child shows a mixture of some of the features of marasmus and kwashiorkor. This is due to the varying nature of the dietary deficiency and the social factors responsible for the disease and presence or absence of infections.

Differences between Kwashiorkor and Marasmus

Kwashiorkor	Marasmus
Kwashiorkor mainly occurs in children in the age group of 1–5 years.	Marasmus occurs in children below the age of 1 year.
It is mainly caused by the deficiency of protein in the diet of child.	It is caused by deficiency of protein as well as carbohydrates in the diet.
The appetite in kwashiorkor is poor.	Appetite is usually good.
In this disease, swelling of body is observed due to oedema (retention of fluids).	No swelling of body takes place in marasmus.
The disease mostly occurs in rural areas where there is small gap period between successive pregnancies.	This disease is more common in towns and cities where breastfeeding is discontinued quite early.
Wasting of muscles is not evident.	In marasmus, wasting of muscles is quite evident. The child is reduced to skin and bones.
Change in the colour of skin occurs in kwashiorkor. The skin becomes scaly in the kwashiorkor.	There is no change in the colour of skin occurs in marasmus. There occurs breaking of skin in marasmus.
The level of serum albumin is low (< 3 g/100 ml blood).	Serum albumin level is normal or sometimes slightly decreased.

Preventive measures

There is no easy solution for the eradication of PEM. There are many strategies which should be adopted for solving the problem of PEM.

According to the 8th FAO/WHO Expert Committee on Nutrition; the following are the ways to prevent:

A. Health promotion

1. Measures directed to pregnant and lactating women (education, distribution of supplements)
2. Promotion of breastfeeding
3. Development of low-cost weaning foods: The child should be made to eat more food at frequent intervals.
4. Measures to improve family diet
5. Nutrition education—promotion of correct feeding practices
6. Home economics
7. Family planning and spacing of births
8. Family environment

B. Specific protection

1. The child's diet must contain proteins and energy-rich foods. Milk, eggs, fresh fruits should be given, if possible.
2. Immunization
3. Food fortification

C. Early diagnosis and treatment

1. Periodic surveillance
2. Early diagnosis of any lag in growth
3. Early diagnosis and treatment of infections and diarrhea
4. Development of programs for early rehydration of children with diarrhea
5. Development of supplementary feeding programs during epidemics
6. Deworming of heavily infested children

D. Rehabilitation

1. Nutritional rehabilitation services
2. Hospital treatment
3. Follow-up care

Nutritional surveillance

Nutritional surveillance comprises the continuous monitoring in a community or area of factors or conditions which indicate the nutritional status of individuals or groups of people. The groups or the individuals who are suffering from the malnutrition must be examined through clinical methods and simple body measurements of the persons who are going for health checkups or attending the health centers. Secondly, the surveys should be done at the regular interval of time and the data must be collected and analysed and then necessary steps should be taken to tackle the problem of malnutrition.

PROGRAMMES FOR ERADICATING MALNUTRITION IN INDIA

Mid-day Meal Scheme

Mid-day meal scheme is also known as National Programme of Nutritional Support to Primary Education, was started on 15th August, 1995 with the goals to enhance enrolment, retention and attendance while simultaneously improving nutritional levels among children in school. It currently covers nearly 12 crore children. The main objectives of the scheme (as per the 2006 revision) are:

- To improve the nutritional status of children in classes one through five in government schools and government aided schools.
- To encourage children from disadvantaged backgrounds to attend school regularly and to help them in concentrating in school activities.
- To provide nutritional support to students in drought-ridden areas throughout summer vacation.

In October 2007 the scheme was revised to cover children in the upper primary section, i.e. the children of classes VI to VII.

Under the scheme a cooked mid-day meal with a minimum of 300 calories and 8–12 grams of protein to all children studying in classes I–V and 700 calories and 20 grams of protein to children of classes VI–VII, by providing grain (rice/wheat) per child/school day.

The central government supplies state and union territory government with free food grains (wheat/rice) at 100 grams per child per school day from the nearest Food Corporation of India (FCI) godown and compensation of the cost of transporting the food grains from the nearest FCI to the Primary school. The scheme provides cooking assistance at the cost of ₹ 1 per child per school day.

Integrated Child Development Services (ICDS)

ICDS comes under Ministry of Social Welfare and was started on 2nd October 1975, for childhood development. The main objective of the programme is to improve the health status of the children and to prevent the causes of child mortality, disability, morbidity and related malnutrition.

Objectives

- To improve the nutritional status of pre-school children of 0–6 years of age group.
- To lay the foundation of proper psychological development of the child.
- To reduce the incidence of mortality, morbidity, malnutrition and school drop out.
- To achieve effective coordination of policy and implementation in various departments to promote child development.
- To enhance the capability of the mother to look after the normal health and nutritional needs of the child through proper nutrition and health education.

The Target Groups

Mainly women and small children are the target of the ICDS programme.

Beneficiaries of the programme	Services provided
Pregnant women	Health check-ups, tetanus toxoid, supplementary nutrition, health education
Nursing mothers	Health check-ups, supplementary nutrition, health education
Children < 3 years	Supplementary nutrition, health check-ups, immunization, referral services
Children between 3 and 6 years	Supplementary nutrition, health check-ups, immunization, referral services, non-formal education
Adolescent girls (11–18 years)	Supplementary nutrition, health education

Components of the scheme

The main components of ICDS are:

Supplementary nutrition: Each child belonging to age group of 6 gets 300 calories and 8–10 g of proteins.

The adolescent girls are given 500 calories and 20–25 g of proteins.

Pregnant and the lactating women are given 500 calories and 20–25 g of proteins.

Malnourished child gets 600 calories and 16–20 g of proteins.

Immunization: Pregnant women and infants are immunized with six vaccines to prevent diseases like poliomyelitis, diphtheria, pertussis, tetanus, tuberculosis and measles.

Referral services: During health check-ups and growth monitoring, sick or malnourished children, in need of prompt medical attention, are referred to the Primary Health Center or its sub-center.

Health check-ups: The height and weight of the children at the regular interval of time is recorded and general check-ups for the detection of the diseases are also done. Prophylactic measures against anemia and vitamin A are also taken.

Adolescent girls scheme (*Kishori Shakti Yojna***):** Under this component, general health check-ups and immunization of adolescent girls are done.

Anganwadi Center: The Anganwadi center delivers the information and services to the families. It is located in the village and is run by Anganwadi worker. The families experiencing the nutrition and health problems contact the Anganwadi worker.

Special Nutrition Programme (SNP)

Another nutritional programme SNP was launched in the country in 1970–71. SNP provides supplementary feeding to the school children and to the expected and nursing mothers. Under this programme about 300 calories and 10 g of protein are provided to preschool children and about 500 calories and 25 g of protein to expect and nursing mothers for six days a week. This programme was operated under Minimum Need Programme. The programme was taken up in rural areas inhibited predominantly by lower socio-economic groups in tribal and urban slums. Fund for nutrition component of ICDS programme is taken from the SNP budget.

Aim of the programme: The main aim of the programme is to improve the nutritional status of the target groups.

Balwadi Nutrition Program

Balwadi refers to a place where, the children in the age group of 2½ to 5 years receive pre-primary education. The balwadi teachers are usually local women.

Activities: In balwadi following activities are carried out:

- Educational activities
- Recreational activities
- Parent teacher meetings
- Nutrition and health awareness
- Medical health check-ups
- Physical education
- Cultural programmes
- Celebration of special events
- Annual day celebration

The *Mahila Mandals* run these balwadis. The children pay a nominal fee through which the teachers' stipend and other expenses are paid. Once the children reach the age of 5, they can be admitted to schools.

Balwadi nutrition programme: Balwadi also runs the nutrition programmes which come under the Department of Social Welfare which are meant for pre-school children. This programme was started in December 1970. The nutritional services are provided to the children in the age group of 3–5 years.

Beneficiaries of the programme: Children belonging to the age group of 3–5 yrs are the beneficiaries.

Supplementary nutrition: Supplementary nutrition of 300 calories and 10 g of protein during 270 days for children attending balwadis are provided.

Allocation of fund: The fund for the supplementary feeding of Balwadi Nutrition Programme is given by the Central Government through voluntary organisations.

Extension of programme: In the present time there are around 5641 balwadis throughout the country benefiting 2.25 lakh children.

STUDY QUESTIONS

1. What is malnutrition?
2. What are the major forms of malnutrition and how is it diagnosed?
3. What are the major components of ICDS programme?
4. Write short notes on:
   a. Mid-day meal scheme
   b. Nutritional surveillance
5. What are the objectives of the nutritional programmes of India?

12 Introduction to Dietetics

INTRODUCTION

In today's era the health problems are the major problems and it is a matter which cannot be ignored. For living a good life health is necessary. Hence, the health professionals are needed at every step of life.

Dietitians and nutritionists are the health professionals who guide, plan, supervise, modify and suggest the diet during the health problems. Dietitians are in a great demand as they do not prescribe any medicines, only the diet is prescribed by them. Diet prescribed by dietitian along with medication helps in improving the health and cures the diseases.

DIETETICS

Dietetics is concerned with planning of diets in maintaining health and in prevention and treatment of disease. It is a science as it uses the rudiments of principles of nutrition and it is an art as it is concerned with the aesthetics of food service.

Objectives of Dietetics

1. To correct the deficiency disorders by solving the dietary problems of the people.
2. To remove hunger and malnutrition prevalent in the society.
3. To help the students in understanding the relationship of health with diet.
4. To improve the quality of life by improving the lifestyle and eating pattern.
5. To make the study advance by introducing the new technical aspect in the field of food and nutrition.

6. To help the government and other health bodies in fighting the health problems.
7. To motivate the students in becoming self reliable and confident.

Career in Nutrition and Dietetics

Dietitian: Dietitian is an expert who plans, supervises, suggests the individuals what to eat or not. They help in modifying the diet if any disease occurs.

Nutritionist: The nutritionist advises about the health in a community. The nutritionist plans and executes the nutritional programmes in the community and helps in improving the health condition in the community.

Who are eligible for the course

The students, who have passed twelfth class with biology and home science with good percentage of marks, can take the admission in the graduate, that is, BSc home science.

For this course they can also pursue a one year diploma course in nutrition and dietetics from a good institute.

Where the demand is more

- In hospitals
- Dairy units
- As consultant
- Day care centers
- Schools and colleges
- As food scientists in big industries and institutions
- In non-governmental organization

Courses offered in dietetics and nutrition

- BSc: Bachelors degree in dietetics and nutrition
- BSc: In clinical dietetics
- BSc: Home science
- Certification course in dietetics and nutrition, diploma in dietetics and nutrition
- PGDND: Postgraduation diploma in nutrition and dietetics
- MSc: Masters of science in dietetics and nutrition

Role of dietitian and nutritionists

1. Dietitian suggests the correct food habits and modifies the diet depending on the severity and demographic condition of the individual.
2. The nutritional value of the foods are evaluated and calculated according to the age, weight, height and deficiency of the individual.
3. The clinical dietitian along with the doctors team plans the diet according to the individual needs.
4. In the food industries they plan and work in improving the quality of food. The microbiological, chemical and nutritional analysis of the food is done.
5. In food product industries they calculate the nutritional values of foods.
6. In the community, dietitians and nutritionists work in the community, public health care centers, social service agencies, *etc.* by providing knowledge regarding healthy food and life style and thus promote good health among the community.
7. The dietitians and nutritionists not only educate, but also train staffs, community and the health care staffs and other employees related with food service department regarding safety and hygiene methods of handling and preparation of food.
8. In the rural areas, various programmes for eradication of malnutrition are running. Hence, by their effective coordination and supervision of the programmes in the community, they can help the government in eradication of malnutrition.

STUDY QUESTIONS

1. What is dietetics? What are its objectives?
2. Who can be a good dietitian? What are the eligibility criteria?
3. What is the role of dietitian and nutritionist in the community?
4. How the nutritionist can eradicate the malnutrition in India?

13 Therapeutic Diet

Diet therapy means use of diet (food and drink) not only in the care of the sick, but also in the prevention of disease and maintenance of health. It is concerned with the use of food as an agent in effecting recovery from illness.

THERAPEUTIC DIET

Therapeutic diets are foods which are given in modified form during the special conditions of lifestyle changes that have strict parameters and a narrow focus. The intention of a diet of this sort is to cleanse, build or increase health following severe illness. Some therapeutic diets could result in vitamin and mineral deficiencies. There are many sustainable, healthy diets that produce holistic results to offset severe illnesses.

Another factor to be considered while planning for therapeutic diet is the diet history. The diet history of the patients help in revealing the patient's past food habits and also his likes and dislikes. The hours of the meal and the economic feasibility should also be considered.

Principles of Therapeutic Diet

The most important principle is to provide all the necessary nutrients so that a good nutritional status is achieved. In the diseased condition, the tissues becomes weak due to inadequacy of nutrients and the essential nutrients are also not utilized. Due to poor utilization of nutrients the digestion becomes difficult and the transportation of nutrients and absorption of the nutrients are also hampered, thus the nutritional status is also hampered.

Thus the diet should be nutritionally adequate and should be modified in such a way that the recovery of the affected part occurs readily and the nutritional requirements of the individual are also met.

Objectives of Diet Therapy

The main objectives of diet therapy are:
1. To maintain a good nutritional status.
2. To correct nutrient deficiencies which have occurred due to the disease.
3. To afford rest to the whole body or to the specific organ affected by the disease.
4. To adjust the food intake to the body's ability to metabolize the nutrients during the disease.
5. To bring about changes in body weight whenever necessary.

The advantages of therapeutic diets are:
1. The psychological and social needs of the individual are met.
2. Food preparation is modified in such a way that family members can modify the meal.
3. The nutritional values are easily calculated.
4. All the essential factors of the diet can be included.

Factors to be considered in planning therapeutic diets:
1. Diseased condition of the individual
2. Duration of the disease

3. Factors and components of the diet
4. Patient's psychological needs
5. Economic status

MODIFICATION OF THERAPEUTIC DIETS

Routine Hospital Diets

1. **Clear liquid diet:** Clear liquid diet is diet without residue and served in fluid form. The diet is non-stimulating, non-irritating and does not form gas. The diet is served in small amounts (usually 30–60 ml) at frequent intervals (2 hr) to replace fluid and electrolytes and to relieve thirst. The diet is mainly composed of water, carbohydrates and some electrolytes provide only 400–500 kcal, 5 g protein, no fat. Clear liquid diet nutritionally inadequate and therefore, used for a very short period of time.

Disease conditions in which the diet is used:
   1. Preoperative patients.
   2. Postoperative patients, e.g. in the initial recovery phase after abdominal surgery or after a period of intravenous feeding.
   3. Endoscopy or colonic examination
   4. Acute illness and infections
   5. As the first step in oral alimentation of a nutritionally debilitated person.
   6. Temporary food intolerance.
   7. During diarrhea or to relieve thirst
   8. For reducing of colonic fecal matter.

2. **Full fluid diet:** Full fluid diet mainly includes the diet which are liquid and is adequately nutritious for patients who cannot chew or who are too ill to do so. It is free from cellulose and irritating condiments and spices. The diet should not be followed for more than two days. This diet is given in between a clear liquid diet and soft diet. The diet provides about 1200 kcal of energy and 35 g of protein. This should be given at 2–4 hr interval.

Disease condition in which the diet are given:
   1. Most often used postoperatively by patients progressing from clear liquids to solid foods.
   2. During acute gastritis and infections.
   3. Oral surgery or plastic surgery of face or neck area.
   4. Chewing and swallowing dysfunction for acutely ill patients.
   5. Esophageal or stomach disorder who cannot tolerate solid foods owing to anatomical irregularity.

3. **Soft diet:** A soft diet is used as a transitional diet between full fluid and normal diet. Soft diet is nutritionally adequate. Soft diet is given in the form of soft food which is seasoned lightly. It is soft in consistency, easy to chew, made up of simple, easily digested foods, containing limited fiber and connecting tissues and does not contain rich or highly flavored foods. The soft diet supplies around 1800 kcal and 50 g protein.

Disease condition in which it is used:
   1. Postoperative patients who are unable to tolerate general diet.
   2. Patients with mild GI problems.
   3. Weak patients or patients with inadequate dentition to handle all foods in a general diet.
   4. Diarrhea convalescence

4. **Mechanical soft diet:** Mechanical diets are prescribed for the people who have lost their teeth. In this diet all the food items in a minced or chopped form can be given.

Disease conditions for its use:
   1. Patients who are unable to chew.
   2. Patients who have undergone head and neck surgery.
   3. Dental problems.
   4. Anatomical oesophageal strictures.

5. **Normal diet:** A normal diet consists of any and all foods eaten by a person in good health. The diet is planned by including all the basic food groups in diet so that optimum amounts of all nutrients are provided. The diet is well balanced and nutritionally adequate. The diet includes the careful attention of dietitian to monitor the food selection and food intake. The RDAs are taken into consideration to achieve the nutritional adequacy. Since the patient is hospitalized or is at bed rest, a reduction and the addition of the nutrients depend on the condition of the patients. The proteins are slightly increased to counteract a negative nitrogen balance. All other nutrients are supplied in normal amounts.

6. **Semi-liquid diets:** This diet is given following tonsillectomy or throat surgery until a soft or general diet may be swallowed without difficulty. It contains cold beverages and lukewarm preparations.

7. **Blenderized liquid diet:** The food items are given in blenderized form and it is given during oral surgery.

SPECIAL FEEDING METHODS

The different modes of feeding patients are:

Enteral
Enteral mode of feeding means, "within or by the way of the gastrointestinal tract." The foods are administered via tube and enteral feeding is also called tube feeding.

Tube feeding
Tube feeding may be advised where the patient is unable to eat but the digestive system is functioning normally. Full fluid diets or commercial formulas may be administered through this route.

Different modes of tube feeding are:

1. *Nasogastric tube feeding:* When the tube is passed through the nose into the stomach.
2. *Nasoduodenal tube feeding:* When the tube is passed through the nose into the duodenum.
3. *Nasojejunal tube feeding:* When tube is passed through the nose into jejunum.

When there is an obstruction in the oesophagus, enteral feeding is done by passing tube surgically through an incision in the abdominal wall into the stomach (gastrostomy), duodenum (duodenostomy) or jejunum (jejunostomy).

Conditions for tube feeding
1. Inability to swallow due to paralysis of muscles of swallowing (diptheria, poliomyelites).
2. Unwillingness to eat.
3. Persistent anorexia requiring forced feeding.
4. Semiconscious or unconscious patients.
5. Severe malabsorption requiring administration of unpalatable formula.
6. Short bowel syndrome.
7. Low birth weight babies.

Parenteral nutrition
In parenteral nutrition, nutrients are delivered directly into the circulation through the peripheral or central vein is termed parenteral nutrition. Intravenous feeding is done in conditions when the patient cannot eat, will not eat, should not eat, cannot eat enough or cannot be fed adequately by tube feeding.

Conditions during which parenteral nutritional occur are:
1. Cancer
2. Inflammatory bowel disease
3. Short-bowel syndrome
4. Preoperative patients
5. Gastrointestinal disorders

Parenteral feed formula
The parenteral feed solutions contain:
- Glucose
- Emulsified fat
- Crystalline amino acids
- Vitamins
- Electrolytes— sodium, chlorine, phosphorus, potassium, calcium and magnesium

- Trace elements—zinc, copper, chromium, manganese and iodine
- Water

Advantages of enteral feeding over intravenous feeding:

1. This is a convenient method of administration of nutrients
2. It is inexpensive.
3. Easily tolerated.
4. No chances of metabolic disturbance

STUDY QUESTIONS

1. What is the importance of therapeutic diet?
2. What are the different types of therapeutic diets?
3. What are the enteral and tube feedings?
4. Write short notes on:
   a. Principles of therapeutic diet
   b. Parenteral feed formula
   c. Diet therapy

14 Diet During Migraines

Migraine is a neurological disorder, often called the severe headache that is believed to occur as a result of complex interactions between the nervous system and the vascular system as well as alterations in brain chemicals.

Types of Migraine

1. **Classic migraine:** A classic migraine is often preceded by warning signs called "aura" (group of symptoms including vision disturbances).
2. **Common migraine:** A common migraine usually comes on without warning.

Causes

Migraine headaches begin during the ages of 10 and 45 years but sometimes they may begin later in life.

The main cause of migraine is the abnormal brain activity. It may also develop due to:

1. Intake of alcohol
2. Anxiety
3. Some odors of perfumes
4. Loud noises
5. Excessive light
6. Changes in hormones during menarche
7. Irregular meals
8. Smoking

Foods responsible for triggering migraine headaches

This can be triggered by common foods such as:

- Processed, fermented, pickled, or marinated foods
- Foods containing monosodium glutamate (MSG)
- Bakery and dairy products
- Foods containing tyramine (**4-hydroxy-phenethylamine**) is a naturally occurring monoamine compound derived from amino acid tyrosine. The chemical acts as a stimulant, leads to headaches and migraines. Foods such as citrus fruits, cheeses, chocolate and alcohol contain tyramine.
- Fruits (avocado, banana, citrus fruit)
- Meats containing nitrates (bacon, hot dogs, salami, cured meats)
- Onions

Symptoms

The most important or the warning sign of migraine is "aura". The aura occurs in both eyes and may involve any or all of the following:

- A temporary blind spot
- Blurred vision
- Eye pain
- Seeing stars or zigzag lines
- Tunnel vision

Other signs include:

1. Difficulty in concentration
2. Nausea
3. Vomiting
4. Fatigue
5. Loss of appetite
6. Numbness, tingling or weakness
7. Sensitivity to light or sound
8. Sweating
9. Neck pain
10. Increased need of sleeping

Tests

Magnetic resonance imaging (MRI) and computed tomography (CT) scans are done for tracing the migraine. A lumbar puncture (spinal tap) might be done.

Treatment

There is no specific cure for migraine headaches. The goal is to treat migraine symptoms and the symptoms can be prevented by adopting good diet and through medication.

During frequent migraines, doctors prescribe medicine to reduce the number of attacks. Antidepressants and blood pressure controlling medicines will help in curing the headaches.

Diet

1. Always take a regular diet. Never skip the food.
2. The diet should be rich in all the nutrients. It should not have the dominancy of one particular nutrient.
3. Breakfast should never be skipped.
4. Take magnesium and riboflavin vitamin supplements regularly. Frequent headaches could indicate you are low in important vitamins and minerals. Low levels of niacin and vitamin B_6, for instance, can cause headaches. Protein-rich foods, like chicken, fish, beans and peas, milk, cheese, nuts and peanut butter are good dietary sources of both niacin and vitamin B_6.
5. The tensions should be avoided and meditations should be done.
6. Meditation is also done.
7. Avoid working for more hours. Take breaks between works.

Foods to be Avoided

Some drinks are known to cause migraine that you could avoid are:
• Red wine
• Champagne
• Drinks containing caffeine like tea, hot chocolate and cola drinks
• Monosodium glutamate, which is present in chinese food as well as many processed foods.
• Nitrates and nitrites present in many cured and processed meats.
• Red wine and cheese.
• Food additives such as aspartame.

Tyramine Containing Foods

Foods such as red wine, aged cheese, smoked fish, chicken livers, figs, and certain beans, chocolates, beans, caffeine, dairy products, soya sauce are the food items which can cause migraine.

STUDY QUESTIONS

1. What is migraine? What are its causes?
2. How foods are responsible for migraine?
3. What are the symptoms of migraine? How can this be treated?
4. What are the dietary considerations during migraines?

15 Diet During Food Allergy

Food is important for growth and for normal functioning of life. But the food may also be responsible for food allergy. Sometimes food when taken not suits the body and presents some characteristics which are problematic and needs attention.

Food allergy is not actually caused by the food but the components which give adverse response to the immune system. The immune system detects the item and when found unhealthy it rejects and some symptoms may develop.

DEFINITION

Food allergy is a hypersensitivity reaction, i.e. it is an abnormal response to a food by our immune system.

Mechanism of Food Allergy

Food allergy is the body's abnormal responses to foods which are not healthy or are harmful. When a person is exposed to the food for which he/she is sensitized, an allergic reaction to an allergen in food can occur. The allergen then stimulates lymphocytes (specialized white blood cells) to produce the immunoglobin E (IgE) antibody that is specific for the allergen. This IgE when released attaches itself to the surface of the mast cells in different tissues of the body. When the individual again eats that particular food, its allergen attaches on the specific IgE antibody on the surface of the mast cells and prompts the cells to release chemicals such as histamine. The various symptoms of food allergy occur when the chemicals are released but all this depends on the types of the tissues in which they are released.

Causes of Food Allergy

One of the most important causes of allergy is the food allergens.

Food Allergens

There are some components which are commonly called food allergens are responsible for causing allergies. These allergens are the proteins which are highly resistant to cooking, acid in the stomach and digestive enzymes. The allergen crosses the gastrointestinal tract and enters into the bloodstream and become the cause of food allergy.

These food allergens can be any edible food or the beverages. Some of the food allergens commonly associated with the food allergy are:

1. Milk is considered as the common allergen. When cow milk is drunk by the children causes allergic conditions because of the presence of casein protein and fails in tolerating the milk and produces allergic symptoms.
2. Wheat flour is also an allergen as it contains gluten which is not digested by some and allergic reactions occur.
3. Eggs are another common food allergen. The egg allergy in some occurs due to the presence of egg white protein while some individuals are allergic to the egg yolk and some people are allergic to both. The individuals who are allergic to egg have an increased risk of developing asthma and nasal allergies.

4. Sea foods such as fishes are also responsible for food allergies.

5. Naturally occurring compounds existing in food sometimes leads to allergy.

It is not necessary that only the foods mentioned above are responsible for food allergy. Anyone having sensitivity of any food item can have the allergy. Allergy can also occur due to ingestion of drugs in contact with food items; common odor such as perfumes, pesticides present in foods, additives, preservatives, trauma and psychological disturbances, tea, coffee, sometimes bacteria and viruses also become the causes of food allergy.

Symptoms of Food Allergy

The symptoms of the food allergy vary with the organ or the part of the body.

Gastrointestinal manifestations: Abdominal pain, nausea, vomiting, diarrhea, gastrointestinal bleeding, colitis, constipation and dyspepsia.

Skin manifestations: Itching, eczema, redness of skin, dermatitis and rashes of the skin.

Respiratory manifestations: Running nose, sneezing, cough, airways obstruction, asthma, and nasal polyps.

Neurologic manifestation: Migraine, neuralgias, tensions, fatigue, anxiety, joints ache

Oral manifestation: Swelling of mouth and throat

Diagnosis

The diagnosis of the food allergy involves the following:

Dietary history

Dietary history is an important tool for diagnosing the food allergy. The doctor asks the questions related to food associated with the allergy and finds the facts. The doctors also ask about the likes and dislikes and then investigate about the symptoms associated with the allergy.

Food diary

Another way of diagnosing the food allergy is keeping the record of the food items daily taken and the timings. The doctors asks the patient to keep the record of his/her meals and to note down the symptoms if occur during intake of the food items. The details help the doctor in diagnosing the food allergy.

Diet elimination

This involves the total restriction of the food items that are suspected to cause allergy.

Skin tests

For detecting the food allergy, some skin tests are also advised by the doctor.

Blood tests

Besides skin tests, blood test is also advised for the confirmation of the food allergy. The blood test measures the presence of food specific IgE antibodies in the blood.

Dietary management in food allergy

The four general principles of allergy management are as follows:

1. The food items which are suspected should be totally avoided.

2. Regular intake of medicines is essential for treating the allergy.

3. Regular check-up is essential.

4. Educate others and be aware before consuming new food.

Diet should be planned well so that the nutritional and caloric needs are well met. The selection of food items should be done carefully and emphasis should be laid on removing the allergy symptoms.

If the food allergy is due to milk, then substitute such as rice milk and other food meeting the nutritional requirements should be selected.

Foods to be included during allergy

The diet should include the hypoallergenic foods. Foods such as rice, beans, pears and apples should be included in the diet.

The foods such as peanuts, millet and wheat need to be avoided as they may cause allergy.

Beverages like rice milk, pear nectar, and clear juice can be useful but sweetener should not be added.

Foods avoided

Wheat, corn, cow's milk, eggs, dairy products, peanuts and soya foods are among the common food allergens, which many times are the cause of food allergy, hence they must be totally avoided.

Sometimes for adding taste and for making meal attractive, artificial food additives are added which often leads to food allergy, hence food containing these chemicals should be eliminated.

STUDY QUESTIONS

1. What is food allergy and what is the mechanism involved?
2. What are food allergens? What are the causes responsible for food allergy?
3. What are the common symptoms occur during food allergy?
4. Write short notes on:
   a. Food allergy
   b. Dietary management in food allergy
   c. Diagnosis of food allergy
   d. Foods to be included

16 Diet During Dental Disorders

Teeth are the very important part of the body which helps in making our body healthy. Our health also depends on the healthy teeth. If the teeth are not healthy, then we cannot eat food and ultimately our health is affected.

Daily we eat a number of food items and the food items which we eat first comes in the contact of the teeth. Healthy eating is thus regarded as important part for the prevention of common dental diseases.

As for living healthy and for normal functioning of the organ, nutrition is important, in the same way caring the teeth is also very essential.

The food item which we eat gets stick to the teeth and if the teeth are not cleaned or not taken care, then disorders may occur. Dental diseases could aggravate to serious conditions like cancerous and infectious ailments.

Today the dental problems are common especially among the children and needs proper attention so that the health is not affected.

Structure of Teeth

The teeth consists of the following parts:

1. **Crown:** Crown is covered with enamel and visible part.
2. **Enamel:** Enamel is the part which covers the crown. This is the hardest substance.
3. **Dentine:** Lines the socket and can be sensitive if the protection of the enamel is lost.
4. **Pulp:** Pulp is the soft tissue having the blood and nerve supply to the tooth.
5. **Cementum:** The layer of bone-like tissue covering the root. It is not as hard as enamel.

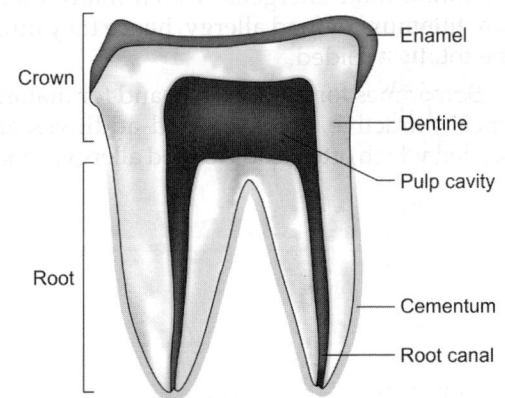

COMMON DENTAL DISORDERS

The most common disorders which occur most are as follows:

1. **Tooth sensitivity:** Tooth sensitivity is the discomfort or pain to one or more teeth or associated areas that are triggered by hot or cold food or even by breathing cold air. Tooth sensitivity mainly occurs due to loss of enamel and cementum which results in exposure of dentin.
2. **Abscessed teeth:** Abscessed tooth is a painful infection at the root of the tooth or between the gums. Abscessed tooth also occurs due to broken or chipped tooth, and gingivitis or gum disease. These problems can cause openings in tooth enamel, which allows bacteria to infect the center of the tooth. The infection can often time spread from the root of the tooth to the bones supporting the tooth.
3. **Stained teeth:** Staining or discoloration of teeth mainly occurs due to food like juice, coffee, tea, cold drinks, wine and even certain antibiotics, can cause the teeth to stain.

4. **Periodontitis or pyorrhea:** Periodontitis is an infection of the ligaments and bones that support the teeth. This occurs due to plaque (plaque is a sticky material made of bacteria, mucus, and food debris that develops on the exposed parts of the teeth) which is not removed from the gums regularly. This causes red gums, or bleeding when you brush or floss.

5. **Gingivitis:** Gingivitis is a form of periodontal disease. This is marked by inflammation and infection that destroy the tissues that support the teeth, including the gums, the periodontal ligaments, and the tooth sockets (alveolar bone). Plaque formation also leads to gingivitis. It is a major cause of tooth decay.

6. **Tooth decay:** Tooth decay is a common disorder. Tooth decay is a common cause of tooth loss and occurs due to the presence of bacteria. These bacteria change sugar and starch into acid and when the acid combines with food pieces and saliva forms plaque which sticks to teeth and decay starts.

CAUSES OF DENTAL DISORDERS

Following are the causes of dental disorders:
- Presence of bacteria in the mouth
- Tobacco
- Misalignment of jaw
- Improper brushing and flossing
- Smoking
- Chewing of toffee and chocolates
- Intake of cold drinks and other carbonated beverages
- Genetic susceptibility

TREATMENT OF DENTAL DISORDERS

1. For treating the dental disorders doctors may prescribe for medicines and antibiotics depending on the disorders and condition of the teeth.
2. For removing bad breath mouth wash is prescribed.
3. Surgery and bone grafts are also done.
4. Fluoride supplements are also effective and they prevent caries.

DIETARY CONSIDERATIONS

The dental problems are mainly linked to fluoride and other mineral deficiencies but diets also play a major role in occurrence of dental disorders.

1. The diet should be rich in vitamins and minerals. A good mineral-rich diet will help in strengthening the tooth.
2. Too much sugar rich foods should not be taken.
3. Confectionary foods such as pasta, rice, potato crisps, fruits, and bread can lead to demineralization of teeth, thus they should not be taken in excess.
4. Lemon and amla are rich sources of vitamin C, thus they must be included in the diet.
5. One should also drink milk regularly as it contains calcium, phosphate and casein, and the milk sugar, lactose, is less cariogenic (caries causing) than other sugars.
6. Fresh yellow-green fruits and vegetables have been identified as beneficial because they are good sources of vitamins A, C and E. Vitamin A is necessary for enamel and vitamin C is essential for dentine.
7. Regular cleaning of mouth and brushing after intake of food also helps in preventing dental disorders.

Tips for Keeping the Teeth Healthy
1. Regular brushing of teeth helps in preventing decaying of teeth.
2. Floss regularly to remove plaque from/ between teeth.
3. Visiting the dentist routinely for a check-up is beneficial.
4. Smoking is also injurious to teeth.

STUDY QUESTIONS

1. What are the common dental disorders which are prevalent in the present time?
2. What are the common causes of dental disorders?
3. What precaution should be taken to prevent dental disorders?
4. What are the dietary considerations which should be followed to prevent dental disorders?

17 Diet During Diarrhea

According to World Health Organization, diarrheal diseases are one of the second leading causes of death in children under 5 years old and every year 1.5 million children die due to diarrhea. The lack of water, salts and gastrointestinal infection are one of the reasons responsible for diarrhea.

DEFINITION

Diarrhea is the passage of loose or watery stools per day, occurring more frequently in the patient than normal individual. Diarrhea is responsible for fluid loss and it could be life taking. Diarrhea is also a leading cause of malnutrition in children under 5 years old. Children with low immunity are at greater risk.

Types of Diarrhea

1. *Acute watery diarrhea*: *Acute diarrhea* is defined as an increased number of stools of decreased form from the normal lasting for several hours and days. If the diarrhea occurs for more than 14 days, it is called *persistent.* If the duration of symptoms is longer than 1 month, it is considered *chronic diarrhea.* Acute diarrhea is caused by microorganisms (e.g. viruses, bacteria, parasites).
2. *Acute bloody diarrhea*: Acute bloody diarrhea or dysentery is caused by bacteria, and is a critical condition. In this type of diarrhea, the blood is mixed with loose, watery stools. The blood mainly comes from digestive tract, or it can come from the mouth and anus. When the diarrhea contains bright red colored blood it is called *hematochezia.*

Causes of Diarrhea

Infection: Diarrhea is caused by rotavirus and bacteria *Escherichia coli* infection. These infections spread through contaminated water.

Malnutrition: Children who die from diarrhea often suffer from underlying malnutrition, which makes them more vulnerable to diarrhea. Each diarrheal episode, in turn, makes their malnutrition even worse. Diarrhea is a leading cause of malnutrition in children under five years old.

Other causes
1. Gastrointestinal surgery
2. Gastrointestinal problems such as ulcers, colitis, *etc.*
3. Allergy and food intolerance to certain foods or medicines.

Complications of Diarrhea

Dehydration: One of the most important complications of diarrhea is dehydration. During diarrhea, due to lack of water important electrolytes such as chloride, sodium and potassium are lost through watery stools, urine and sweat.

During severe dehydration death may also occur.

Signs of dehydration
1. Inelastic skin
2. Dry lips and mouth
3. Furred tongue
4. Sunken fontanelle (the soft spot on a baby's head)
5. Weakness

Treatment of Diarrhea

One of the important goals of treatment is to improve the condition of the patient by giving adequate amount of fluids.

- *Rehydration*: With intravenous fluids in case of severe dehydration or shock and/or oral rehydration salts (ORS) solution for moderate or no dehydration. ORS is a mixture of clean water, salt and sugar, which can be prepared safely at home. It costs a few cents per treatment. ORS is absorbed in the small intestine and replaces the water and electrolytes lost in the feces.
- *Zinc supplements*: For reducing the duration of diarrhea and for reducing the stool volume, zinc supplements are necessary.
- *Nutrient-rich foods*: As malnutrition may lead to diarrhea, thus for treating the malnutrition, the diet should be nutritionally adequate and it should include a variety of nutritious foods.

Prevention of Diarrhea

Diarrhea can be prevented by:

1. Keeping the environment clean
2. Exclusive breastfeeding for the six months
3. Maintaining proper hygienic condition
4. Vaccination
5. Health education

Work of WHO

WHO along with his members works as:

- Promote current policies for the management of diarrhea in developing countries.
- Conduct research to develop and test new health delivery strategies in this area.
- Develop new health interventions, such as the rotavirus immunization.
- Help to train health workers, especially at community level.

Diet In Diarrhea

Dietary Modifications

The most important aim of treating the diarrhea is the management of fluid and electrolyte balance.

Management of Fluids

The loss of body fluids should be replaced by a liberal intake to prevent dehydration. Water, fruit juice, vegetable soups, rice kanji with salt, fresh lemon with sugar or honey can be given.

Electrolytes

During diarrhea electrolytes such as sodium and potassium are lost which leads to weakness. For electrolytes ORS solution in small sips should be taken regularly.

Energy

In acute diarrhea over 1500 kcal daily and in chronic diarrhea about 2500 kcal are given.

Proteins

The diet should contain protein-rich foods. The protein-rich foods which can be easily digested should be given.

Fats

The diet having fats should be restricted as they may aggravate diarrhea.

Fiber

A low fiber diet is suggested for diarrheal patients.

Foods to be Avoided

Food items such as spices, pulses, fried foods and fibrous vegetables should be avoided.

Diet in Chronic Diarrhea

Low milk, milk free and starch free diet can be given as represented in table:

Type of diet	Composition
Diet A/Level I diet	Low milk diet (50 ml/kg/day) curd, rice with milk.
Diet B/Level II diet	Milk free diet—cereal—pulse mix/amylase rich foods.
Diet C/Level III diet	Lactose—Sucrose/starch free diet soya based or chicken based, and egg.

Source: Elizabeth KE 2002. Nutrition and child development, Paras publishing, Hyderabad and Bangalore.

Weanling Diarrhea

The diarrhea occurs in very small children during introduction of weaning food. During weaning the infant's digestive system is not mature as there occurs no secretion of enzymes which are essential for digestion.

Dietary Management

Small children having diarrhea may lead to protein energy malnutrition, thus the diet should include easily digestible protein-rich foods.

The following points should be considered for managing diarrhea in small children:

- The infant should be breastfed regularly.
- Better hygienic conditions should be adopted.
- Small children may develop protein energy malnutrition hence, they must be given protein-rich foods in diet.
- ORS solution in small sips should be given at regular interval of time.
- Cereals and pulse mixture can be given.
- Banana in mashed form can be given.

Prevention

a. The foods which are sold on the roadside or which are exposed to flies should not be taken.

b. The food items before cooking should be washed carefully and should be cooked well.

c. The utensils should be carefully washed and should be kept at a clean place.

d. The kitchen should be cleaned and mopped regularly by using disinfectant.

e. The fruits should be washed and peeled before consumption.

f. Water should be drink at regular interval of time.

STUDY QUESTIONS

1. What is diarrhea? How it occurs?
2. What complications occur during diarrhea?
3. What is ORS? Define its composition.
4. Discuss the following:
   a. Diet during diarrhea
   b. Diet in weanling diarrhea

18 Diet in Burns

In our day-to-day life we often met with accidents such as we fall from stairs or we often get burn during cooking food or while walking in the sun. Burns happen when our skin exposes to heat from fire, electricity, sun (UV rays) or it may be pouring of hot liquids on the body surface. Burns damage our outer skin and lead to damage of our nerves.

TYPES OF BURNS

Burns are classified into 3 categories:

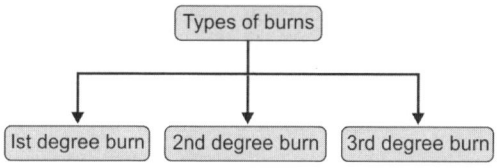

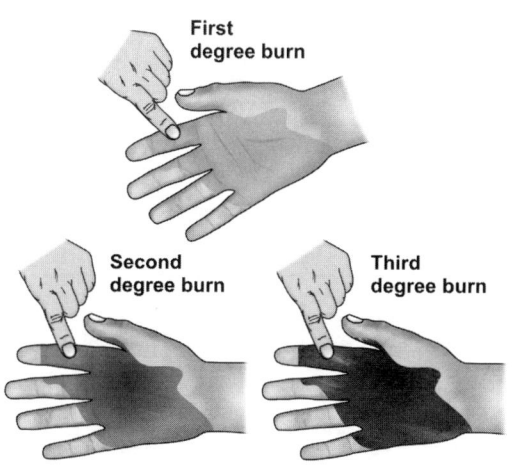

1. **1st degree burn:** In first degree burns, only the outer layer—epidermis damages. These burns are treated by themselves. Cold water gives relief.

2. **2nd degree burn:** In these, the damage to the lower layer of the skin occurs. The blisters occur and if they are not broken the injured area remains protected.

3. **3rd degree burn:** The subcutaneous layer is affected and need medical attention. The third degree burn is dangerous. The blood loss may affect the circulation and the dehydration may also occur.

Complications
- When the burns are severe, extensive fluid loss may occur and severe tissue damage occurs
- Dehydration
- Damage of muscles and blood vessels
- Infections
- Respiratory problems

Treatment
1. For first degree burn:
   a. Wash under running cool water
   b. Ibuprofen or acetaminophen to relieve pain and swelling
2. For second degree burn:
   a. Wash under running cool water
   b. Ibuprofen or acetaminophen to relieve pain and swelling
   c. Do not break the blisters

3. For third degree burn:
   a. When the clothes stuck to the skin, do not remove it.
   b. Wash under running cool water.
   c. Cover the burned area with a sterile bandage or a clean sheet.
   d. Do not apply any ointment.

Diet in Burns

Principle of the Diet

A high calorie, high protein for tissue formation with healing of wounds and with vitamins and minerals are necessary for the patients suffering with burns.

The diet of the patient should be rich in antioxidants and fluids and should be taken at regular interval of time.

Proteins

For the recovery of wounds and for the formation of new tissues the diet should contain adequate amount of proteins. According to nutrition experts the diet should contain 1.5–2.5 of the proteins per kg body weight. Foods such as milk and its products, pulses and eggs should be included in the diet to meet the protein requirements.

Carbohydrates

For meeting the energy requirement of burn patient, a high carbohydrate diet is essential. Foods such as rice, bread, potatoes, sugar and corn should be included in the diet to meet the energy requirements.

Fat

For increasing calories and adding bulk in diet, fat is necessary. Butter, oil and cream should be taken in the diet.

Vitamins and Minerals

Vitamin needs increase for the repairment of the tissues and for normal functioning of the tissues. Vitamin C is essential for healing the wounds and for collagen synthesis. For therapeutic purposes, vitamin B complex is needed.

STUDY QUESTIONS

1. How burn occurs?
2. What are the major categories of burns?
3. What complications occur during burn? How are they treated?
4. What type of diet should be given to the burn patients?

19 Diet in Diabetes Mellitus

Diabetes is considered as a major healthcare problem in India. According to Diabetes Atlas published by the International Diabetes Federation (IDF), there were an estimated 40 million persons with diabetes in India in 2007 and this number is predicted to rise to almost 70 million people by 2025. The countries with the largest number of diabetic people will be India, China and USA by 2030. It is estimated that every fifth person with diabetes will be an Indian. Due to these sheer numbers, the economic burden due to diabetes in India is amongst the highest in the world.

According to ICMR India based study new figures for diabetes prevalence in India indicate that the epidemic is progressing rapidly across the nation, reaching a total of 62.4 million persons with diabetes in 2011. The study concludes that in India about 62.4 million people live with diabetes and 77.2 million people are on the threshold, with pre-diabetes.

WHAT IS DIABETES MELLITUS?

Diabetes mellitus is a group of metabolic diseases which occurs due to insufficient secretion of insulin. Diabetes is characterized by increased level of blood sugar.

Insulin is a hormone secreted by β cells of islets of Langerhans of pancreas.

Functions of Insulin

Insulin has the following functions:
- It causes the cells in the liver, muscle and fat tissue to take up glucose from blood and convert it to glycogen that can be stored in the liver and muscles.

- Insulin also prevents the utilization of fat as an energy source. In absence of insulin glucose is not taken up by body cells, and the body begins to use fat as an energy source.
- Insulin also helps in regulating the amino acid uptake by body cells.

The blood glucose levels are controlled by insulin. Insulin lowers the blood glucose level. When the elevation in blood glucose occurs (for example, after eating food), insulin is released from the pancreas to normalize the glucose level. In patients with diabetes, the absence or insufficient production of insulin causes hyperglycemia (high blood sugar). Diabetes is a chronic medical condition, meaning that although, it can be controlled, it lasts a lifetime.

Types of Diabetes

Type 1 Diabetes

Type 1 diabetes is also called insulin dependent diabetes mellitus (IDDM) or Juvenile diabetes. As the name Juvenile, it mainly occurs in children and adolescents. In IDDM, there is a little or no production of insulin and as a result, such individuals require daily insulin injections. There is usually a sudden onset. When the injections are discontinued, the symptoms become more severe.

Type 2 Diabetes

Type 2 diabetes is also referred to as non-insulin dependent diabetes mellitus (NIDDM), or adult onset diabetes mellitus (AODM). In type 2 diabetes, the insulin is produced in deficient amount. While it is often initially managed by increasing exercise and dietary modification, medications are typically needed as the disease progresses.

Malnutrition Related Diabetes Mellitus (MRDM)

MRDM is mainly seen in India. It occurs in young people between 15 and 30 years of age. The people suffering with MRDM are lean and undernourished. In this type of diabetes, the pancreas fails to produce adequate insulin. As a result, these diabetics require insulin.

Gestational Diabetes

Gestational diabetes occurs during pregnancy. During pregnancy, the hormonal changes make cells less responsive to insulin. During pregnancy, sometimes the increased insulin demand cannot be fulfilled and the blood sugar level rises too high and results in gestational diabetes.

Risk Factors for Diabetes

1. *Hereditary*: The risk of a child developing diabetes with a parental history increases above 50 percent. A high incidence of diabetes is seen among the first degree relatives.

2. *Obesity*: The chances of diabetes in obese individuals is 3 times higher than in non-obese individuals. People with high waist circumference are at greater risk of having diabetes mellitus. Waist circumference expands with increasing body waist. If waist circumference is greater than normal, then the chances of diabetes are increased.

3. *Physical inactivity*: The individual who does not take exercise, becomes obese which ultimately leads to diabetes. Physically inactive individuals have a 40% chance of developing diabetes mellitus.

4. *Undernutrition*: Lack of nutrients leads to undernutrition which impairs β-cell function by increasing the susceptibility of individuals to genetic and environmental influences.

5. *Stress*: Stress precipitates diabetes in susceptible individuals. In stress, the body releases adrenaline, noradrenaline, cortisone that raises blood glucose levels and counteracts available insulin. During stress, blood glucose may rise and ketosis may occur.

6. *Intake of alcohol*: Heavy intake of alcohol may lead to hypoglycemia and intolerance to glucose.

Symptoms

Polydipsia (excessive thirst)

Polyphagia (increased appetite especially for sweets)

Polyuria (frequent urination)

Itching

Easy tiring, weakness or irritability

Drowsiness

Slow healing of cuts and wounds

Frequent infections of the skin, gums and vagina and pain in the legs, feet, urinary tract or fingers

Blurred vision

Weight loss

Hyperglycemia (elevated blood sugar level) above 140 mg/100 ml, the normal level being 80–100 mg/100 ml — a deficient supply of functioning insulin affects the metabolism of carbohydrates, fats and proteins. As a consequence, glucose enters to the circulation and hyperglycemia follows.

Glycosuria (sugar in the urine)

Diagnosis

Oral Glucose Tolerance Test (OGTT)

In OGTT, 12 hours of overnight fasting is done. About 75 g of glucose in adults and 1.75 g/kg of body weight in children is orally administered. Before the administration of glucose and after two hours, blood samples are collected and glucose levels are checked. In a person with diabetes, the fasting blood glucose concentration is almost always above 110 mg/100 ml and often above 140 mg/100 ml.

The blood sugar levels increase after the glucose load and come down to basal level within two hours.

Benedict's Test

In this test, about 8–10 drops of Benedict's reagent is added in 5 ml of urine. It is then boiled for two minutes or placed in a boiling water bath for three minutes. It is then allowed to cool spontaneously. A precipitate forms varying from greenish to yellowish brown to reddish brown, roughly according to the amount of reducing substance present. A white precipitate may be produced, if considerable amounts of phosphates are present. Positive results are obtained, if reducing substances equivalent to more than 0.10 to 0.15 percent of glucose, by blood sugar methods, are present.

It is better to carry out this test on the second urine sample collected in the morning as urine sugar in this sample will more or less reflect blood sugar level.

DIETARY MANAGEMENT

Diabetes can be treated by diet alone, or diet and hypoglycemic drugs or diet plus insulin depending on the type and severity of the condition.

Points to be remembered for treating diabetes:
1. Reduction of sugar in blood and urine
2. Maintaining the ideal body weight
3. Taking a balanced diet
4. Making diet healthy with emphasis on reducing the sugars

Energy

The calculated calorie requirement should allow the patient to lose or gain weight as required and maintains body weight 10% lower than the ideal / desirable body weight. Dietary calories should be 60–70 percent from carbohydrate 15–20 percent from protein and 15–25 percent from fat. The recommended calorie intake for a diabetic based on body weight is as follows:

Overweight individual— 20 kcal/kg wt/day

Ideal weight— 30 kcal/kg wt/day

Underweight— 40 kcal/kg wt/day

Carbohydrate

High carbohydrate helps in insulin binding. For carbohydrates, the diet containing cereals and pulses are given. These are then broken down into simple sugars before they are absorbed from the gut. Refined carbohydrates such as sugar, honey, jaggery and jam contain simple sugars which are directly absorbed are not recommended for diabetics, as they cause a rapid rise in blood sugar. Sugar present in fruits and milk raise the blood sugar at a slightly lower rate. Whole apple is better than apple juice because of its high fibre content.

Protein

It is recommended that 15–20% of total calories be derived from proteins. Proteins supply essential amino acids needed for tissue repair. Proteins do not raise blood sugar during absorption and do not supply as many calories as fats. In patients with NIDDM, consumption of protein along with carbohydrate will lower the blood glucose concentration. One gram of protein per kilogram body weight is adequate.

Fat

Diet with low fat diet helps in increasing insulin binding and also reduces LDL (low density lipoprotein) and VLDL (very low density lipoprotein) levels and reduces the incidence of atherosclerosis which is more common in diabetics. Fat content should be 15–25% of total calories and higher in polyunsaturated fatty acids.

Vitamins

Vitamin A
Vitamin A is necessary for healthy vision and prevents blindness.

Food sources: Food sources of vitamin A include liver, eggs, fish liver oil and β-carotene as its biological precursor is found in carrots and other orange coloured vegetables.

Vitamin B Complex

Vitamins B_1, B_2, B_3, B_5, B_6, B_{12} and folic acid are necessary for metabolic functions. They are important for the body's energy metabolism, which involves the utilisation of glucose as energy source, the conversion of glucose and for mobility of stored energy into glucose.

Food sources: Food sources of B-vitamins include whole grain cereals, pulses, dairy products, eggs and dark green leafy vegetables.

Vitamin C

Vitamin C, also known as ascorbic acid is a very important antioxidant. Vitamin C is important for the maintenance of healthy connective tissues and is important for healing of tissues and prevents damage of the circulatory system.

Food sources: Food sources of vitamin C include citrus fruits, sweet peppers, chillies, guavas, lettuce and tomatoes.

Vitamin E

Vitamin E is another important antioxidant vitamin. Vitamin E plays a very important role in the maintenance of the circulatory system, in support of healthy blood circulation.

Food sources: Dietary sources of vitamin E include amla, wheat germ, nuts and seeds.

Minerals

Magnesium

Magnesium is a mineral which is required in the body for the transport of glucose across cell membranes and therefore, plays an important role in diabetic control. With poorly controlled diabetes and subsequent frequent urination, magnesium is lost through the urine, which may result in magnesium deficiency. Patients with Type 2 diabetes have been shown to have lower levels of magnesium. Magnesium deficiency is associated with hypertension and changes in blood lipids, which relate to an increased risk for cardiovascular disease.

Food sources: Broccoli, peas, spinach and other dark green leafy vegetables contain magnesium. Other food sources include lean red meat and whole grain cereals.

Zinc

Zinc is a mineral with antioxidant properties that play a role in numerous enzyme functions of the body. Zinc deficiency is associated with impaired blood glucose control as well as impaired wound healing, which already is a problem for most diabetics. Therefore, zinc as mineral is not only important for blood glucose control in the body, but also for wound healing. Zinc also plays an important role in the healthy functioning of the immune system and is an essential nutrient for eye health.

Food sources: Sea food, especially shellfish such as oysters are rich in zinc. Other food sources include pumpkin seeds, sunflower seeds, pulses and eggs.

Other food sources: Food sources include carrots, spinach, butternuts and pumpkins.

Dietary fibre

Intake of 25 g of dietary fibre per 1000 calories is considered optimum for a diabetic. High fibre foods have a low caloric value and therefore, diabetics should consume such foods liberally. Fibre present in vegetables, fruits, legumes and fenugreek seed is soluble in nature and more effective in controlling blood sugar and serum lipid than insoluble fibre present in cereals.

Exercise

Regular exercise should be an integral part of the daily routine of the diabetic.

Patient Education

Having knowledge regarding diabetes is beneficial for the diabetics. Diabetics should be educated regarding diabetes and its consequences. They must be told about the dietary concepts and should be encouraged to follow a healthy diet with regular intake of medicines and exercise should be taken daily to ensure overall well being. Adequate information enables the diabetics to improve the psychological acceptance of the disease. They must be informed about the symptoms of hypoglycemia and the immediate need for sugar. The body weight should be measured regularly and if any complications arise, they must consult their doctor.

STUDY QUESTIONS

1. What is diabetes and what is the role of insulin in body?
2. Discuss about the types of diabetes.
3. What are the major risk factors associated with diabetes?
4. How the diabetes will be diagnosed?
5. Write notes on:
   a. Diet in diabetes
   b. Patient education

Appendices

Food Exchange List

Vegetable Exchange A

These vegetables may be used as desired. Carbohydrates and calories are negligible.

Leafy vegetables	Other vegetables
Amaranth	Drumstick
Bathua	French beans
Brussels sprouts	Knol-Khol
Cabbage	Ladiesfingers
Celery	Mango, green
Coriander leaves	Onion stalks
Curry leaves	Parwar
Fenugreek leaves	Plantain flower
Lettuce	Pumpkin
Mint	Raddish
Rape leaves	Rhubarb stalks
Spinach	Snake gourd
Soya leaves	Tinda
	Tomato, green
	Turnip
	Ridge gourd
	Snake gourd

Vegetable Exchange B

Carbohydrates— 10 g, Calories— 50 kcal
Root vegetables

Food	Quantity (g)
Beetroot	75
Carrot	105
Colocasia	45
Onion (medium)	90
Potato	45
Sweet potato	30
Tapioca	30
Yam	45

Other Vegetables

Food	Quantity (g)
Artichoke	60
Broad beans	90
Cluster beans	90
Double beans	50
Jack, tender	105
Jackfruit seeds	30
Leeks	60
Peas	45
Plantain, green	75

Fruit Exchange

Carbohydrates— 10 g, Calories— 50 kcal

Fruit quantity (gm) approximate number of size

Foods	Quantity (g)	Number of size
Amla	90	Medium
Apple	75	Small
Banana	30	Medium
Gooseberry	150	Small
Cashew fruit	90	Medium
Custard apple	50	–
Dates	30	–
Figs	135	Medium
Grapes	105	–
Grape fruit	150	Big
Guava	100	Medium
Jackfruit	60	Medium pcs.
Jambu fruit	50	Big
Lemon	90	Medium
Mango	90	Small
Melon	275	Medium
Orange	90	Small
Papaya	120	Medium
Peach	135	Medium
Pear	90	Medium

Contd.

Fruit quantity (gm) approximate number of size (Contd.)

Foods	Quantity (g)	Number of size
Pineapple	90	Slices (round)
Plum	120	Medium
Pomegranate	75	Small
Strawberry	105	–
Sweet lime	150	Medium
Tomato	240	Medium
Watermelon	175	Small

Cereal Exchange

30 g provide calories: 100 kcal
Carbohydrates: 20 g; protein: 2 g

Bajra	Rice flakes
Barley	Rice puffed
Bread*	Sago**
Jowar	Samai
Cornflakes	Semolina
Maize, dry	Vermicelli (savian)
Oatmeal	Wheat flour
Ragi	Wheat, broken (dalia)
Rice	White flour

*To meet carbohydrates and calories add 5 g sugar

**Requires supplementation with other high protein foods, when used

Legume and Pulse Exchange

30 g provide calories: 100 kcal
Carbohydrates: 15 g; protein: 6 g

Bengal gram	Kabuli Channa (White gram)
Bengal gram,	Roasted Lentils
Black gram, Cow gram	Peas, dried
Green gram	Rawan
Horse gram	Red gram

Flesh Food Exchange

Calories: 70 kcal; protein: 10 g

Food	Quantity (g)
Beef 60	60
Crab 120 g	120
Egg, duck* 2 Nos.	2 Nos.
Egg, hen* 2 Nos.	2 Nos.
Fish, big 60	60
Fish, small 60	60
Fish, vajra 60	60

Contd.

Contd.

Food	Quantity (g)
Fowl 60	60
Liver, sheep 60	60
Mutton muscle* 60	50
Pigeon 50	60
Pork 60	60
Prawn 60	

* Provides 100 calories

Milk Exchange

Calories 100 kcal; protein 5 g

Food	Quantity
Butter milk	750 ml
Cheese	30 gm
Curd	210 gm
Khoa	30 gm
Milk, buffalo	90 ml
Milk, cow	180 ml
Milk, skimmed	260 ml
Milk, skimmed powder*	30 gm

* Provides 10 g protein

Fat Exchange

Calories: 100 kcal; Fat: 11 g

Food	Quantity (g)
Almonds	15
Butter	15
Cashewnuts	20
Coconut	30
Ghee	11
Groundnuts	20
Hydrogenated fat (vanaspati)	11
Oil (coconut, mustard)	11
Pistachionut	15
Walnuts	15

APPENDIX B

Revised recommended dietary allowances for Indians — 2010

Group	Category	Body wt.		Energy (kcal/Day)		Proteins (g/day)		Visible fat (g/day)	
		Revised	Old	Revised	Old	Revised	Old	Revised	Old
	Sedentary	60	60	2320↓	2425			25↑	
Man	Moderate			2730↓	2875	60	60	30↑	22
	Heavy			3490↓	3800			40↑	
	Sedentary			1900	1875			20	
Woman	Moderate			2230	2225			25↑	20
	Heavy	55↑	50	2850↓	2925	55↑	50	30	
	Pregnant			+350↑	+300	78↑	65	30	30
	Lact. <6 mths			+600↑	+550	74	75	30↓	45
	Lact. 6–12 mths			+520↑	+400	68	68	30↓	
	0–6 mths	5.4	–	92/kg↓	108/kg	1.16/kg↓	2.05/kg	–	–
Infants	6–12 yrs	8.4	8.6	80/kg↓	98/kg	1.69/kg	1.65/kg	19	–
	1–3 yrs	12.9	12.6	1060↓	1240	16.7↓	22	27	
Children	4–6 yrs	18.0	19.0	1350↓	1690	20.1↓	30	25	25
	7–9 yrs	25.1	26.9	1690↓	1950	29.5↓	41	30↑	
Boys	10–12 yrs	34.3	35.4	2190	2190	39.9↓	54	35↑	22
Girls	10–12 yrs	35.0	31.5	2010↑	1970	40.4↓	57	35↑	
Boys	13–15 yrs	47.6	47.8	2750↑	2450	54.3↓	70	45↑	22
Girls	13–15 yrs	46.6	46.7	2330↑	2060	51.9↓	65	40↑	
Boys	16–17 yrs	55.4	57.1	3020↑	2640	61.5↓	78	50↑	22
Girls	16–17 yrs	52.1	49.9	2440↑	2060	55.5↓	63	35↑	

Revised recommended dietary allowances for Indians — 2010

Group	Category (µg/day)	Calcium		Iron (mg/day)		Retinol (µg/day)		β-carotene (mg/day)	
		Revised	Old	Revised	Old	Revised	Old	Revised	Old
	Sedentary								
Man	Moderate	600↑	400	17↓	28	600	600	4800↑	2400
	Heavy								
	Sedentary								
Woman	Moderate	600↑	400	21↓	30	600	600	4800↑	2400
	Heavy								
	Pregnant	1200↑	1000	35↓	38	800↑	600	6400↑	2400
	Lact. <6 mths								
	Lact. 6–12 mths	1200↑	1000	21↓	30	950	950	7600↑	3800
	0–6 mths		–	46 µg/kg	–				
Infants	6–12 yrs	500	500	5	–	350	350	2800↑	1200
	1–3 yrs						12		
Children	4–6 yrs	600↑	400	13↓	18	400	400	3200↑	1600
	7–9 yrs			16↓	26	600	600	4800↑	2400
Boys	10–12 yrs	800↑	600	21↓	34				
Girls	10–12 yrs			27↑	19				
Boys	13–15 yrs	800↑	600	32↓	41	600	600	4800↑	2400
Girls	13–15 yrs			27	28				
Boys	16–17 yrs	800↑	500	28↓	50				
Girls	16-17yrs			26↓	30				

Revised recommended dietary allowances for Indians — 2010

Group	Category	Thiamine (mg/day)		Riboflavin (mg/day)		NiacinEq. (mg/day)		Vitamin B$_6$ (mg/day)	
		Revised	Old	Revised	Old	Revised	Old	Revised	Old
	Sedentary	1.2	1.2	1.4	1.4	16	16		
Man	Moderate	1.4	1.4	1.6	1.6	18	18	2.0	2.0
	Heavy	1.7	1.6	2.1↑	1.9	21	21		
	Sedentary	1.0	0.9	1.1	1.1	12	12		
Woman	Moderate	1.1	1.1	1.3	1.3	14	14	2.0	2.0
	Heavy	1.4↓	1.2	1.7↑	1.5	16	16		
	Pregnant	+0.2	+0.2	+0.3	+0.2	+2	+2		
	Lact. <6 mths	+0.3	+0.3	+0.4	+0.3	+4	+4	2.5	2.5
	Lact. 6–12 mths	+0.2	+0.2	+0.3	+0.2	+3	+3		
	0–6 mths	0.2	55 µg/kg	0.3	65 µg/kg	710 µg/kg	710 µg/kg	0.1	0.1
Infants	6–12 yrs	0.3	50 µg/kg	0.4	60 µg/kg	650 µg/kg	650 µg/kg	0.4	0.4
	1–3 yrs	0.5↓	0.6	0.6	0.7	8	8	0.9	0.9
Children	4–6 yrs	0.7↓	0.9	0.8	1.0	11	11		
	7–9 yrs	0.8↓	1.0	1.0	1.2	13	13	1.6	1.6
Boys	10–12 yrs	1.1	1.1	1.3	1.3	15	15	1.6	1.6
Girls	10–12 yrs	1.0	1.0	1.2	1.2	13	13		
Boys	13–15 yrs	1.4↑	1.2	1.6↑	1.5	16	16		
Girls	13–15 yrs	1.2↑	1.0	1.4	1.2	14	14	2.0	2.0
Boys	16–17 yrs	1.5↑	1.3	1.8↑	1.6	17	17		
Girls	16–17 yrs	1.0	1.0	1.2	1.2	14	1		

Revised recommended dietary allowances for Indians — 2010

Group	Category	Vitamin C (mg/day)		Dietary folate (µg/day)		Vitamin B$_{12}$ (µg/day)		Other Minerals	
		Revised	Old	Revised	Old	Revised	Old	Zinc (mg/day)	Mg (mg/day)
	Sedentary								
Man	Moderate	40	40	200	100	1	1	12	340
	Heavy								
	Sedentary								
Woman	Moderate	40	40	200	100	1	1	10	310
	Heavy								
	Pregnant	60↑	40	500	400	1.2↑	1		
	Lact. <6 mths	80	80	300	150	1.5	1.5	12	310
	Lact. 6–12 mths								
	0–6 mths							–	30
Infants	6–12 yrs	25	25	25	25	0.2	0.2	–	45
	1–3 yrs			80	30			5	50
Children	4–6 yrs	40	40	100	40	0.2–1.0	0.2–1.0	7	70
	7–9 yrs			120	60			8	100
Boys	10–12 yrs	40	40	140	70	0.2–1.0	0.2–1.0	9	120
Girls	10–12 yrs								160
Boys	13–15 yrs	40	40	150	100	0.2–1.0	0.2–1.0		165
Girls	13–15 yrs								210
Boys	16–17 yrs	40	40	200	100	0.2–1.0	0.2–1.0		195
Girls	16–17 yrs								235

Source: Dr. Brahmam GNV Scientist– 'F', HOD Division of community studies, National Institute of Nutrition, (ICMR) Jamai-Osmania (PO), Hyderabad

APPENDIX C

Websites

http://www.drugswell.com/wow/index.php

http://wiki.answers.com

http://www.umm.edu/

http://www.askdrsears.com/html/4/T041300.asp

http://health.nytimes.com/health/guides/nutrition/vitamin-e/overview...

http://www.textbooksonline.tn.nic.in

http://www.umm.edu

http://www.medicalcriteria.com

http://education.nic.in/mdm/mdm2004.asp

http://www.foodallergy.org/

www.vrg.org/veg/

www.who.org/nut

APPENDIX D

Glossary

Abscess: Swollen, inflammed, tender area of infection filled with pus.

Absorption: Transfer of nutrients across cell membranes following digestion, nutrients are transferred from the intestine to the blood and lymph circulation.

Acidosis: The condition which occurs due to accumulation of an excess of acids in the body, or by excessive loss of minerals cations form the body.

Achalasia: Condition of the esophagus that disrupts normal swallowing.

Acute: Beginning suddenly. Severe but of short duration.

Adenosine triphosphate (ATP): A compound containing one molecule of adenine and ribose and three molecules of phosphoric acid: two phosphate groups are held by high energy bonds.

Adrenal: Pertaining to one or both glands located adjacent to the kidneys. These glands secrete many hormones, including adrenalin, and play an important part in the body's endocrine system.

Adrenal cortex: Outer layer of the adrenal gland. Secretes various hormones including cortisone, estrogen, testosterone, cortisol, androgen, aldosterone and progesterone.

Aldehydes: A large group of compounds containing the group –CHO

Aldosterone: A steroid hormone produced by the adrenal cortex.

Amine: Organic chemical compound containing nitrogen.

Amylase: An enzyme that hydrolyzes starch, e.g. ptyalin

Anaphylaxis (Allergic shock): Severe, life-threatening allergic response to medications or other allergy-causing substances.

Androgenic arrhenoblastoma: Ovarian

Anemia: Condition in which the number of red blood cells or hemoglobin (oxygen carrying substance in blood) are inadequate.

Anorexia: Loss of appetite

Antibody: A protein substance produced in an organism as a response to the presence of an antigen mainly as defense mechanism.

Antigen: Any substance produced in an organism as a response to the presence of an antigen mainly as a defense mechanism.

Antibiotic: A substance produced by living organism that inhibits the growth of other organisms, used as a food preservative in some countries.

Anthocyanin: Water soluble pigment of many fruits, flowers, leaves and roots, which changes colour from red, violet to blue, depending on acidity.

Antioxidants: Substances that prevent cell damages and prevent free radical formation.

Anuria: Lack of urinary secretion.

Ascites: Accumulation of fluid in the abdominal cavity.

Aseptic: It is a method of handling, in which entry of microorganisms in food is prevented.

Atrophy: Wasting away; diminishing in size such as a cell, tissue, organ or part. May result from disease, lack of use, aging or other influences.

Autoimmune: Response directed against the body's own tissue.

Autoimmune disease: Disease in which the immune system produces antibodies that attack the body's own tissues.

Basal energy expenditure: The amount of energy used in 24 hours by a person who is lying quietly, 12 hour after the last meal, in a comfortable temperature and environment.

Beriberi: A deficiency disorder which occurs due to deficiency of thiamin characterized by polyneuritis, edema (in some cases), enlargement of heart and rapid heartbeat.

Bilirubin: Yellowish red blood cell waste product in bile the blood carries to the liver. It contributes to the yellow color of urine. Can cause jaundice if it builds up in the blood. Formed mainly by the breakdown of hemoglobin in red blood cells after the end of their normal life span.

Biopsy: Removal of a small amount of tissue or fluid for laboratory examination; aids in diagnosis.

Blanching: Dipping of fruits or vegetables in boiling water or exposing these to steam for a few minutes to kill enzymatic and biological activity prior to freezing or processing.

Blood: Liquid pumped by the heart through arteries, veins and capillaries. It consists of a clear, yellow fluid called plasma and formed elements of cells. Blood's major function is to transport oxygen and nutrients to cells and remove carbon dioxide from cells and other waste products for detoxification and elimination.

Blood corpuscles: Red Blood Cells (RBCs) and White Blood Cells (WBCs)

Body Mass Index (BMI): Body Mass Index is a standardized ratio of weight to height, and is often used as a general indicator of health. BMI can be calculated by dividing weight (in kilograms) by the square of your height (in metres).

Bone marrow: Specialized soft tissue that fills the core of bones. Most of the body's red and white blood cells are produced in bone marrow.

Botulism: It is a food poisoning caused by toxins secreted by *Clostridium botulinum*.

Buffer: Substance which resists change in pH (alkalinity and acidity).

Calorie: Calorie is a unit of measurement for energy. One calorie is formally defined as the amount of energy required to raise one cubic centimetre of water by one degree centigrade. One kcal is also equivalent to 4.184 kilojoules.

Caries: Decaying of teeth

Calcification: It is a process by which an organic tissue becomes hard by deposition of calcium salts.

Capillary: A minute blood vessel connecting the small arteries (arterioles) and small veins (veniules). The exchange of materials between the blood and tissues takes place through the walls of the capillaries.

Carnitine: An amino acid which forms an ester with fatty acetyl COA to facilitate the transfer of long-chain fatty acids across mitochondrial membranes for oxidation.

Capillary: A minute blood vessel connecting the small arteries (arterioles) and small veins (venules). Exchange of materials between the blood and tissues takes place through the walls of the capillaries.

Carotenoids: Group of fat-soluble, yellow orange plant pigments.

Carrier: A person in apparent good health, who harbors pathogenic microorganisms and passes these on to others.

Catalyst: A substance which increases the rate of a chemical reaction without being used up in the reaction.

Cell: The smallest structural and functional unit of plant and animal organisms.

Cholecystitis: Gallbladder inflammation usually caused by a gallstone that cannot pass through the cystic duct.

Cholesterol: A fat produced by liver and is essential for normal functioning of body.

Chronic: Long-term; continuing. Chronic illnesses are usually not curable, but they can often be prevented from worsening. Symptoms usually can be controlled.

Cirrhosis: Inflammation and scarring of liver tissues resulting in impaired liver function.

Coenzyme: A coenzyme is a cofactor which is needed by enzymes for a biochemical change.

Cofactor: A non-protein chemical compound bounded to protein required for the protein's biological activity.

Colitis: Inflammatory condition of the large intestine. It can occur in episodes, such as irritable bowel syndrome, or it can be one of the more serious, chronic, progressive, inflammatory bowel diseases, such as ulcerative colitis. See ulcerative colitis. Irritable bowel syndrome is characterized by bouts of colicky abdominal pain, bloating, diarrhea or constipation, and fatigue, often due to emotional stress. Treatment includes stress reduction, diet changes and sometimes medication.

Conjunctiva: A fine membrane covering eyeball and lining or gaseous phases.

Colostrum: First fluid, i.e. milk secreted after the child is born.

Congenital: Present at, and existing from, the time of birth.

Congestive heart failure: Complication of many serious diseases in which the heart loses its full pumping capacity. Blood backs up into other organs, especially the lungs and liver.

Contamination: Entry of microorganisms in food items.

Copper: Copper is a trace element that is essential for absorbing and utilizing iron.

Cyst: Sac or cavity filled with fluid or disease matter.

Cystic fibrosis: Inherited disease in which mucus-producing glands throughout the body, especially in the pancreas and lung, fail to produce normal enzymes and mucus.

Cytotoxic: Having a negative effect upon cells.

Deficiency: Lack of nutrients.

Dehydration: Loss of water from the body, which is not compensated by intake of water.

Dementia: A mental disorder occurring due to impaired transfer of nerve impulses.

Denaturation: Structural changes in proteins due to effect of heat, light and change in pH. Changes in solubility also occur.

Dialysis: Process of separating crystals and other substances in a solution by the difference in their rate of diffusion through a semipermeable membrane.

Dietary fiber: Plant fibers that include cellulose, hemicellulose, lignin, gums and pectin.

Diffusion: Movement of molecules from high concentration to lower concentration.

Digestion: Mechanical and chemical breakdown of food to simple substance which can be absorbed and used by the body cells.

Disease: Process representing a departure from normal health.

Diverticulitis: Inflammation of diverticula. During periods of inflammation, person experiences crampy pain and fever. White blood cells increase to fight off infection.

DNA: Deoxyribonucleic acid helps in formation of genetic material.

Disaccharide: Carbohydrate that consists of two monosaccharide units.

Duodenum: First portion of small intestine.

Duodenal ulcer: Peptic ulcer located in the duodenum, which is the first segment (about 10 inches long) of the small intestine that leads from the stomach.

Dwarfism: Underdevelopment of the body.

Dysentery: Inflammation of the intestine, especially the colon; may be caused by chemical irritants, bacteria, viruses, parasites or protoza. Characterized by frequent, bloody stools, abdominal pain and ineffective painful straining to have a bowel movement (tenesmus).

Dyspnea: Difficulty breathing.

Essential amino acids: Essential amino acids (EAA) are not synthesized by our body. EAA are—histidine, isoleucine, leucine, lysine, methionine, phenylalanine, theronine, tryptophan, and valine are considered essential, since they must be supplied by our diet.

Edema: Accumulation of fluid under the skin (swelling), in the lungs or elsewhere.

Enteritis: Inflammation of the mucous membrane lining of the small intestine.

Esophageal varices: Enlarged veins on the lining of the esophagus subject to severe bleeding. They often appear in patients with severe liver disease.

Esophagus: Hollow tube that provides passage from the back of the throat to the stomach.

Essential fatty acids (EFA): Fatty acids which the body needs, but cannot be synthesized. The two main EFAs are linoleic acid and linolenic acid.

Exudate: Matter that penetrates through vessel walls into adjoining tissue. Production of pus or serum. Accumulation of fluid in a cavity.

Fetal hypoxia: Absence of sufficient oxygen to sustain life in a fetus.

Fibrosis: Formation of fibrous tissue in repair process.

Fibrin: Protein formed from fibrinogen by the action of blood clotting.

Fibroids: Abnormal growth of cells in the muscular wall of the uterus (myometrium). Uterine fibroids are composed of abnormal muscle cells and are almost always benign. Cause is unknown. Usually decreases in size without treatment after menopause.

Fibromas: Benign neoplasm of fibrous or fully developed connective tissue.

Flavonoids (bioflavonoids): Flavonoids are a class of water-soluble pigments that are found in many plants. They also serve as antioxidants.

Gallstones: Calculus or stone formed in the gallbladder.

Gastrin: Hormone that stimulates the production of gastric acid or stomach acid.

Gastritis: Irritation, inflammation or infection of the stomach lining. Cause is sometimes unknown but may be due to excess stomach acid, food allergy, viral infection or adverse reaction to alcohol, caffeine or some drug. Symptoms may include nausea, diarrhea, abdominal pain, cramps, fever, weakness, belching, bloating and loss of appetite.

Gastroenteritis: Inflammation of the stomach and intestines accompanying many digestive-tract disorders. Causes may include bacterial, viral or parasitic infections, food poisoning, food allergy, excess alcohol consumption or emotional upset.

Gastrointestinal disease: Any disorder of the gastrointestinal tract, which includes the mouth, esophagus, stomach, duodenum, small intestine, cecum, appendix, the ascending colon, transverse colon, descending colon, sigmoid colon, rectum and anus.

Gastrointestinal disorders: Any condition or disease relating to any part of the digestive system, including the mouth, esophagus, stomach, small intestine, large intestine and rectum. May also include some conditions relating to the liver, gallbladder and pancreas.

Gastrointestinal (GI) symptoms: Any symptoms relating to the stomach or intestine. Some common GI symptoms include vomiting, diarrhea, constipation, bloating and heartburn.

Glaucoma: Abnormally increased pressure within the eyeball that may produce severe, permanent vision defects. It is the most preventable cause of blindness. If diagnosed and treated early, it rarely results in permanent loss of vision.

Glycogen: Substance formed from glucose, stored chiefly in the liver. When the blood sugar level is too low, glycogen is converted back to glucose for the body to use as energy.

Goiter: Enlargement of the thyroid gland, which causes a swelling in the front part of the neck.

Gout: Recurrent attacks of joint inflammation caused by deposits of uric acid crystals in the joints. It can be very painful.

Growth spurt: The period of growth when the growth rate is fastest.

Haemorrhoids: Commonly known as piles.

Haematuria: Condition in which urine contains blood.

Hemolytic jaundice: Jaundice caused by severe hemolytic anemia, which results in high levels of unconjugated bilirubin. Leads to a jaundiced appearance. See bilirubin, unconjugated; anemia, hemolytic; jaundice.

Hemorrhoids: Dilated (varicose) veins of the rectum or anus. Usually caused by straining during bowel movements, although pressure from a rectal tumor or pregnancy may cause them. Symptoms may include rectal bleeding, pain, itching or mucus discharge after bowel movements and a lump that can be felt in the anus. If hemorrhoids are very large, there may be a sensation that the rectum has not emptied completely after a bowel movement.

Hepatic: Of or affecting the liver.

Hepatic coma: Stupor or coma caused by waste products in the blood that are toxic to the brain. Normally, waste products are neutralized by the liver, but due to extensive liver damage they continue to circulate in the blood. Can cause death.

Hereditary: Transmitted genetically from generation to generation.

Hydrocephalus: Condition characterized by an excessive accumulation of fluid with the cranial vault.

Hyper: Abnormally increased; excessive.

Hypertension (high blood pressure): Increase in the force of blood against the arteries as blood circulates through them. Often has no symptoms. Essential or primary hypertension, the most common kind, has no single identifiable cause. Secondary hypertension is caused by an underlying disease.

Hyperthyroidism: Overactivity of the thyroid, an endocrine gland that regulates all body functions.

Hypertonic: Solution that contains substances that flow outward through a semipermeable membrane into a solution of lower concentration.

Hypertrophy: Increase in the size of a cell or group of cells. Causes an increase in the size of an organ or part.

Hypo: Deficient; beneath; under.

Idiopathic: Without known cause.

Immunodeficiency diseases: Defects in the body's immune system. A healthy immune system protects the body against germs (bacteria, viruses, fungi), cancer (partial protection) and any foreign material that enters the body. When the system fails, the body becomes susceptible to infection and cancer. Can range from minor to very severe.

Infant mortality rate: Number of infant deaths in the first year of life per 1000 live births.

Infarction: Tissue death due to the obstruction of blood to that tissue.

Influenza: Common, contagious respiratory infection caused by a virus. Incubation after exposure is 24 to 48 hours.

Insulin: Hormone secreted by beta cells of the islet of Langerhans.

Intravenously (IV): Through a vein.

Invisible fats: Fat present as an integral component of plant and animal foods such as in cereals and legumes.

Iron overload: Too much iron in blood, liver or other organs.

Ischemia: Decreased blood supply to a body organ or part.

Ischemic: Condition in which there is decreased blood flow to a body organ or part.

Ischemic bowel disease: Intestinal problems caused by inadequate supply of blood to the cells of the intestines.

Jaundice: Condition of yellow skin, yellow whites of the eyes, dark urine and light-colored stools. It is a symptom of diseases of the liver and blood caused by abnormally elevated amounts of bilirubin in the blood.

Keratosis: Any horny growth, such as a wart.

Ketogenesis: Synthesis of ketones.

Ketone bodies: Substances formed when the body rapidly breaks down fats to use for energy.

Ketonemia: Presence of ketones in the blood.

Ketonuria: Presence of ketone bodies in the urine. Usually seen in people with uncontrolled diabetes mellitus or as a result of starvation.

Ketosis: Condition resulting from incomplete oxidation of fatty acids, and the consequent accumulation of ketones like acetone, beta-hydroxybutyric acid and aceto acetic acid.

Kilocalorie: The amount of heat required to raise the temperature of 1 kg of water by 1 °C.

Lactational amenorrhea: Cessation of monthly menstrual period during the period of lactation.

Lactic acidosis: Increased acidity in body due to accumulation of excessive lactic acid production.

Larynx: Part of the air passage connecting the throat with the trachea or windpipe.

Lesion: Injury or damage to an organ or tissue.

Leukemia: Blood cancer

Luteum: Yellow-colored cyst.

Lymph: Transparent, slightly yellow liquid found in lymph vessels throughout the body. Derived from tissue fluids.

Lymphatic: Pertaining to lymph system of the body.

Lymphatic system: Vast, complex network of vessels, valves, ducts, nodes and organs that help protect and maintain the internal fluid environment of the body. Responsible for transporting fats, proteins and other substances to the bloodstream. Lymph glands produce antibodies that help fight infections.

Lymphocyte: One of the several types of white blood cell that help fight infection.

Lymphoma: Disorders involving new, abnormal growth or tumor of lymph tissue. Usually malignant but may be benign. Usually afflicts men.

Lysis: Destruction or breakdown, as of a cell or other substance.

Macroamylaemia: Excess of starch in the blood.

Malignant: Capable of causing destruction of normal tissue; may lead to death. Usually refers to cancer growth.

Mast cells: Part of connective tissue.

Medulla: Most internal part of a structure or organ.

Meninges: Thin membranes that cover the brain and spinal cord.

Meningitis: Inflammation or infection of the meninges.

Menarche: The onset of menses in females.

Menopause: Permanent cessation of menstruation. Occurs as early as age of 35 or as late as age of 55; usually spans 1 to 2 years. Menopause is only one event in the *Climacteric*, a biological change in body tissue and body systems that occurs in both sexes between the mid-40s and mid-60s.

Menstrual: Pertaining to menstruation.

Metabolism: Sum of all the chemical and physical processes by which living substance is produced and maintained. Also includes the concept of the transformation by body cells by which energy is made available.

Muscular dystrophy: Gradual deterioration of the muscles of the body, leading to increasing difficulties in walking and moving.

Myocardial fibrosis: Formation of fibrous material in the heart.

Myocardial infarction (heart attack): Death of heart muscle cells from reduced or obstructed blood flow through the coronary arteries.

Myocardium: Heart muscle.

Necrosis: Localized death of tissue that occurs in groups of cells in response to disease or injury.

Nephritis: Inflammation of the nephrons

Nephrosis: Degeneration of the nephrons.

Neuritis: Inflammation of a nerve.

Nocturia: Urination at night.

Nutrient balance: The balance between intake and output for a particular nutrient.

Obstructive jaundice (cholestasis): Interruption in the flow of bile through any part of the biliary tract. Causes can occur in or outside the liver.

Occlusion: Closing or obstruction. Usually describes a blockage in blood vessels.

Oedema: Abnormal accumulation of fluid in the intercellular tissue spaces or body cavities.

Oliguria: Scanty secretion of urine.

Osmolarity: It is a measure of the osmotically active particles per liter of the solution. It is expressed as mOsm/l.

Osmotically: It is a measure of the osmatically active particles per kilogram of the solvent in which the particles are dispersed. It is expressed as mOsm/kg.

Osteomalacia: Abnormal condition resulting in softening of bone. Accompanied by weakness, fracture, pain and weight loss. May be caused by a diet lacking in phosphorus, calcium or vitamin D, lack of exposure to sunlight or malabsorption.

Osteopenia: A metabolic bone disease common in preterm infants, also called rickets of prematurity.

Osteoporosis: Loss of normal bone density, mass and strength, leading to increased porousness and vulnerability to fracture. Usually occurs in women after menopause. Treatment includes a well-balanced, nourishing diet, specific vitamin-mineral supplements, exercise and sometimes estrogen replacement.

Pancreatitis: Inflammation of the pancreas. Chronic pancreatitis usually follows recurrent attacks of acute pancreatitis. Pancreas gradually becomes unable to supply digestive juices and hormones necessary for good health.

Parasites: Organisms that live within, upon or at, the expense of another living organism. Human parasites include disease-causing agents, such as amoebas or worms, that infect the digestive system or fungi that live on skin.

Parathyroids: Small glands that control calcium levels in the blood and bones. Located within or next to the thyroid gland in the lower neck, next to the trachea.

Pathology laboratory: Laboratory where tissues, blood, urine, feces and other parts of the human body are studied to determine cause of disease.

Peptic ulcer: Lesion of the mucous membrane lining of the stomach, duodenum or of any part of the digestive tract exposed to stomach acids. Acute peptic ulcers are often shallow and cause no scars or symptoms. Chronic peptic ulcers are often deep, cause scarring of the tissue and are persistent.

Pericardium: Thin, membranous, double-layered covering of the heart.

Phlebitis: Inflammation of a vein.

Plaque: Any patch area: Atherosclerotic plaque is a deposit of lipid material in the blood vessel.

Plasma: Fluid part of the blood after blood cells and other particles are removed.

Plasmin: Active portion of the chemical system that causes blood clots to dissolve.

Pneumonia: Inflammation of the lung(s) resulting in tiny air sacs in the lung becoming plugged with exudate. Can be caused by bacteria, viruses or fungi.

Polycystic: Containing many cysts.

Polycythemia: Increase in red blood cells in the body. The disease has three forms. Polycythemia vera involves overproduction of red blood cells, white blood cells and platelets. Secondary polycythemia is a complication of diseases or factors other than blood cell disorders. Stress polycythemia involves decreased blood plasma.

Polyps: Growths. Often on a stalk arising from dry mucous membranes, such as in the nose, cervix or colon.

Prophylaxis: Prevention of disease

Proteinuria: Excretion of protein in the urine

Pulmonary: Lungs

Purging: The use of self-induced vomiting, laxatives or diuretics to prevent weight gain.

Purpura: Purplish or brownish discoloration easily seen through the skin caused by bleeding into the tissues.

Radiography: Making X-ray films of internal structures of the body by exposure of film specially sensitized to X-rays or gamma rays.

Renal: Pertaining to the kidney.

Renal plasma flow: Rate of blood flow through the kidney.

Reflux esophagitis: Irritation of the esophagus from stomach acid splashing upward into the esophagus.

Rickets: Condition caused by insufficient intake or absorption of vitamin D coupled with too little exposure to sunlight. Seen primarily in infants and small children.

Rooting reflex: If the baby's cheek is touched, the baby will turn towards that side.

Retina: Innermost part of the eyeball.

Salmonella: Thousand kinds of salmonella bacteria cause many diseases, including typhoid fever, paratyphoid fever and some forms of gastroenteritis (inflammation of the stomach and intestines.

Satiety: Satiety refers to the feeling of satisfaction or "fullness" produced by the consumption of food.

Scan: A diagnostic procedure using a scintillation camera to record images of various parts of the body following injection of appropriate radioactive substances. This is a major tool for establishing precise diagnoses.

Scurvy (Vitamin-C deficiency): Illness caused by inadequate intake of vitamin C. Vitamin C is essential for the body to manufacture connective tissue (collagen) that helps to form healthy bones, teeth and capillaries, and promotes wound healing. Symptoms in children may include tender, swollen legs, bleeding and bruising under the skin, bleeding gums, fever and anemia. See Anemia. Adults may have swollen, bleeding gums, tooth loss, bleeding or bruising under the skin or bleeding into joints, weakness and mental changes.

Serum: Liquid portion of the blood that remains after blood cells have been removed.

Shigellosis: Dysentery produced by an infection by a shigella germ.

Spina bifida: Inherited defective closure of the body encasement of the spinal cord through which the cord and meninges may protrude.

Staphylococcus aureus: Bacteria that frequently causes diseases of the skin and other organs.

Sterol: A sterol is any of a class of solid cyclic alcohols, found in both plants (e.g. campesterol, stigmasterol, beta-sitosterol) and animals (e.g. cholesterol).

Syndrome: Set of symptoms that occur together.

TSH (Thyroid-stimulating hormone): Chemical substance secreted by the pituitary gland; controls the release of thyroid hormone from the thyroid gland. TSH is needed for normal thyroid growth and function.

Tachycardia: Heartbeat that is too fast.

Thrombosis: Blood clot in a blood vessel.

Transamination: The reversible transfer of an amino group from an amino acid to a keto acid, forming a new keto acid and a new amino acid without the appearance of ammonia.

Tuberculosis: Contagious, bacterial infection caused by the germ mycobacterium tuberculosis. Usually affects the lungs, but may spread to other organs.

Ulcer: Round, crater-like lesion of the skin or mucous membrane resulting from tissue death. Accompanies some inflammatory, infectious or cancerous conditions.

Uremia: Presence in blood of excessive amounts of protein metabolism byproducts, such as urea.

Ureter: Tube that carries urine from the kidney to the bladder.

Urethra: Hollow anatomical structure that leads from the bladder to outside the body.

Urethritis: Inflammation or infection of the urethra.

Urogenital: Referring to the kidney and reproductive systems of the human body. Also called genitourinary.

Varices: Enlarged veins, arteries or lymph vessels.

Vasopressin: Also called anti-diuretic hormone. Hormone made by the hypothalamus and stored in the pituitary gland. Effects include contraction of the muscular layer of small blood vessels, contraction of the smooth muscles of the intestinal tract and stimulation of contraction of the uterus.

Visible fats: Fats and oils that can be used directly or in cooking.

Xerophthalmia: Abnormal dryness and thickening of the mucous membrane lining of the eyelids and white part of the eye and cornea. Occurs due to deficiency of vitamin A.

APPENDIX E

One Word Questions

1. An electron carrier in the mitochondrial electron transport chain of the cell, having antioxidant properties in vitro

Ans. Ubiquinone

2. Ubiquinone is synthesized in the body from precursor of

Ans. Cholesterol

3. The component which plays an important role in the aetiology of oedema in kwashiorkor

Ans. Copper

4. Antioxidant which has been found in maintaining memory

Ans. Vitamin C

5. The component which has been found useful in progression of moderately severe Alzheimer's disease

Ans. β-tocopherol

6. Cognitive ability is supported by

Ans. Vitamin B_6 and vitamin B_{12}

7. The vitamin which has been found to prevent oxidation of PUFA in cell membranes

Ans. Vitamin E

8. Chewing of betel nuts leads to loss of vitamin

Ans. Thiamine (Vitamin B_1)

9. Pellagra is caused by the deficiency of

Ans. Niacin (Vitamin B_2)

10. The important proteins present in meat are

Ans. Actin, myosin, collagen and elastin

11. Oils and fats give about _____ kcals of energy/100 gms.

Ans. 900 kcals

12. Spices and condiments have _____ properties.

Ans. Anticarcinogenic

13. Biomedically health is _____

Ans. Freedom from all diseases

14. Lack of essential nutrients in the diet leads to _____ .

Ans. Malnutrition

15. For nourishment and disease-free life, _____ diet is necessary.

Ans. Balanced diet

16. According to ICMR there are _____ essential food groups.

Ans. Five

17. For growing child the diet should contain good quality _____ rich foods.

Ans. Protein

18. Vitamin C is necessary for preventing _____ .

Ans. Scurvy

19. Vitamin _____ is necessary for reproduction.

Ans. Vitamin E

20. Protein is regarded as _____ .

Ans. Body building foods

21. _____ is the energy giving component of food.

Ans. Carbohydrates

22. Term vitamin was coined by

Ans. Funk

23. _____ are regarded as the poor sources of energy.

Ans. Vitamins

24. Thiamine is

Ans. Vitamin B_1

25. _____ is the good source of vitamin C.

Ans. Amla

26. The vitamin which is not present in vegetables is

Ans. Vitamin D

27. Cod liver oil is a very good source of

Ans. Vitamin D

28. The vitamin necessary for blood clotting is

Ans. Vitamin K

29. _____ is regarded as the necessary component for teeth

Ans. Calcium

30. Spinach is good source of _____

Ans. Iron

31. Besides carbohydrate and protein, milk is also a good source of

Ans. Calcium and potassium

32. _____ is important for preventing anemia.

Ans. Iron

33. In typhoid, _____ is effected.

Ans. Intestine

34. The bacteria responsible for typhoid is

Ans. _Salmonella typhi_

35. Rickets occur due to deficiency of

Ans. Vitamin D

36. _____ is required for the synthesis of RNA and DNA.

Ans. Folate

37. _____ is also important for synthesis of collagen.

Ans. Vitamin C

38. For mineralization of bones _____ is essential.

Ans. Calcium and phosphorus

39. For proper digestion _____ is essential.

Ans. Water

40. Children should not be motivated to eat _____

Ans. Junk foods

41. For nitrogen equilibrium, intake of _____ is essential.

Ans. Protein

42. Normal level of hemoglobin in female is _____ /100 ml.

Ans. 12–13 g

43. Deficiency of iron leads to _____

Ans. Anemia

44. For the formation of new bones of the growing fetus _____ is essential.

Ans. Calcium

45. Calcium requirement of adult woman is _____

Ans. 400 mg/day

46. Iron store after birth of child last for _____

Ans. 4–6 months

47. For preventing constipation during pregnancy _____ rich diet should be taken.

Ans. Fiber

48. _____ is a carbohydrate which is stored in liver.

Ans. Glycogen

49. _____ is also a fiber.

Ans. Cellulose

50. _____ is a polysaccharide.

Ans. Chitin

51. Gliadin and zein are the proteins mainly found in _____

Ans. Wheat

52. The movement of muscles occur due to presence of _____ and _____ proteins.

Ans. Actin and myosin

53. The _____ enzyme is essential for breakdown of proteins.

Ans. Pepsin

54. _____ hormone stimulates protein production in muscle cells.

Ans. Somatotropin

55. _____ hormone helps in contraction of uterus muscles during child birth.

Ans. Oxytocin

56. Hair and nails are made of _____ protein.

Ans. Keratin

57. _____ is necessary for transportation of oxygen in the body.

Ans. Hemoglobin

58. Each gram of proteins provides _____ kcal of energy.

Ans. 4 kcal

59. _____ is a very rich source of protein.

Ans. Soyabean

60. Besides carbohydrates, _____ are also considered as source of energy.

Ans. Fat

61. Vitamin K is essential during pregnancy for preventing _____ among neonates.

Ans. Hemorrhage

62. For flushing out the toxins _____ should be taken regularly.

Ans. Water

63. _____ are the proteins which are present in bones.

Ans. Glycoproteins

64. Two or more proteins are joined by a _____ linkage.

Ans. Peptide

65. _____ hormone is essential for maintaining blood glucose level in the body.

Ans. Insulin

66. 1 gram of proteins gives about _____ kcal of energy.

Ans. 4 kcal

67. LDL is also known as _____

Ans. Bad cholesterol

68. Chemical name of vitamin B_5 is _____.

Ans. Pantothenic acid

69. _____ is the energy reservoir of glycogen in animals and plants.

Ans. Glycogen

70. Potato is a rich source of _____ .

Ans. Starch

71. In the absence of oxalo acetic acid _____ is converted into ketone bodies.

Ans. Acetate

72. _____ adds bulk to the diet and helps in stimulation of peristaltic movements.

Ans. Cellulose

73. _____ is a important constituent of bile acids and a precursor of vitamin D.

Ans. Cholesterol

74. The deficiency of vitamin B_2 leads to dry chapped appearance of the lips which is also known as

Ans. Cheilosis

75. LDL is _____ which is also called

Ans. Low density lipoprotein, bad cholesterol

76. _____ is necessary for formation of new DNA.

Ans. Niacin

77. Pantothenic acid, i.e. vitamin B_5 is also known as _____

Ans. Antistress vitamin

78. _____ is essential for the production of RNA and DNA.

Ans. Vitamin B_9 (Folic acid)

79. For increase in appetite _____ is essential.

Ans. Cyanocobalamin (Vitamin B_{12})

80. For preventing the growth of microorganisms, canning is done at _____ this temperature.

Ans. 100 °C

81. _____ and _____ are the food items which are sun dried.

Ans. Papad and mango

82. _____ is a preservative which are added in tomato and grape juices.

Ans. Sodium benzoate

83. Consumption of khesari dal leads to

Ans. Lathyrism

84. Iodine is required for the synthesis of _____ and _____ hormones.

Ans. Triiodothyronine (T_3) and thyroxine (T_4)

85. _____ are the special types of rays used to preserve the food.

Ans. Gamma rays

86. Electric oven is used for _____ the foods.

Ans. Baking

87. Earthen oven is also known as _____

Ans. Tandoor

88. _____ is a combined method of roasting and stewing.

Ans. Braising

89. On exposure to heat the green color of green leafy vegetables changes to _____

Ans. Olive green color

90. PEM is _____

Ans. Protein energy malnutrition

91. The deficiency of protein and energy in the diet results in _____

Ans. Protein energy malnutrition

92. _____ and _____ are the forms of PEM.

Ans. Kwashiorkor and marasmus

93. Kwashiorkor is also known as _____

Ans. Malignant malnutrition

94. _____ occurs due to lack of energy and protein in the diet.

Ans. Marasmus

95. BUN stands for _____

Ans. Blood urea nitrogen

96. For improving the nutritional status of children _____ programme was started.

Ans. Mid-day-meal programme

97. ICDS stands for _____

Ans. Integrated child development services

98. Special nutrition programme was launched on _____

Ans. 1970–71

99. The increase in cholesterol level may lead to _____

Ans. Athreosclerosis

100. *Aspergillus flavus* secretes

Ans. Aflatoxin

101. _____ is concerned with planning of diets.

Ans. Dietetics

102. _____ is diet in modified form

Ans. Therapeutic diet

103. The objective of therapeutic diet is to _____

Ans. Maintain good nutritional status

104. Planning of diet involves calculation of _____

Ans. Nutritive values

105. _____ diet is used only for a short period of time.

Ans. Clear fluid diet

106. Full fluid diet provides about _____ of calorie.

Ans. 1200 kcal

107. Patients with mild gastrointestinal problems are often given _____ diet.

Ans. Soft

108. The diet in which foods are given in minced and chopped form is known as _____

Ans. Mechanical diet

109. The word enteral means _____

Ans. Within or by way of gastrointestinal tract

110. The process in which nutrients are delivered directly into the circulation through the peripheral or central vein is termed _____

Ans. Parenteral nutrition

111. The big advantages of enteral feeding is that _____

Ans. This is a convenient method of administration of nutrients

112. _____ is a neurological disorder which is also called severe headache.

Ans. Migraine

113. MRI is expanded as _____

Ans. Magnetic resonance imaging

114. _____ is a naturally occurring monoamine compound derived from amino acid tyrosine which acts as stimulant, leads to headaches and migraines.

Ans. Tyramine

115. The abnormal response to a food by our immune system is known as _____

Ans. Food allergy

116. Food allergy can be diagnosed by _____

Ans. Dietary history

117. _____ is a painful infection at the root of the tooth or between the gums.

Ans. Abscessed tooth

118. _____ is a common cause of dental disorders.

Ans. Improper brushing

119. For preventing scurvy _____ rich foods should be included in diet.

Ans. Vitamin C

120. An increased number of stools of decreased form from the normal lasting for several hours and days is _____ form of diarrhea.

Ans. Acute

121. When the diarrhea contains bright red colored blood it is called _____

Ans. Hematochezia

122. _____ is most important complications of diarrhea.

Ans. Dehydration

123. ORS is _____

Ans. Oral rehydration solution

124. The diarrhea which occurs in small children during introduction of weaning food is termed _____

Ans. Weanling diarrhea

125. When the subcutaneous layer is harmed during burn, this burn is _____

Ans. 3rd degree burn

126. For better recovery of wounds _____ are essential.

Ans. Proteins

127. Vitamin C is essential for _____

Ans. Wound healing

128. The word lipos means _____

Ans. Fat

129. The increase in cholesterol level may lead to _____

Ans. Atherosclerosis

130. _____ vitamin is good for health of dentine.

Ans. Vitamin C

131. The major cause of anemia in our country is _____

Ans. Lack of iron in diet

132. The metabolic disease which occur due to insufficient secretion of insulin _____

Ans. Diabetes

133. _____ is a hormone secreted by α cells of islets of Langerhans of pancreas.

Ans. Insulin

134. The levels of blood glucose is maintained by _____

Ans. Insulin

135. Type 1 diabetes is also known as _____

Ans. Insulin dependent diabetes mellitus (IDDM) or juvenile diabetes

136. Type 2 diabetes is also referred to as _____

Ans. Non-insulin dependent diabetes mellitus (NIDDM), or adult onset diabetes mellitus (AODM)

137. MRDM is _____

Ans. Malnutrition related diabetes mellitus

138. Diabetes occurring during pregnancy is called _____

Ans. Gestational diabetes

139. Hyperglycaemia is _____

Ans. Increased blood sugar level

140. For diagnosing diabetes _____ tests are carried out.

Ans. OGTT (oral glucose tolerance test) and Benedict's tests

141. Low intake of fat helps in _____

Ans. Reducing the risk of cardiovascular diseases

142. The intake of vitamin A helps the diabetics in reducing

Ans. Deterioration of eyesight

143. Magnesium is necessary for reducing the incidence of _____

Ans. Hypertension

144. Fenugreek seeds should be taken by diabetic because they are good sources of _____

Ans. Fiber

145. Proteins help in _____

Ans. Maintenance of tissue repair

146. Vitamin C is necessary for _____

Ans. Healing of tissues

Bibliography

American Heart Association Nutrition Committee; Lichtenstein AH, Appel LJ, Brands M, *et al.* Diet and lifestyle recommendations revision: A scientific statement from the American Heart Association Nutrition Committee. *Circulation*; 114:82–96, 2006.

Bamji Mehtab S, *et al.* (ed). Textbook of Human Nutrition, Oxford & IBH Publishing Co. Pvt. Ltd., New Delhi, 1998.

Corinne Robinson, Marilyn H, Lawler R. Normal and Therapeutic Nutrition, Oxford & IBH Publishing Co. New Delhi, 1982.

Dowd P, Hershline R, Ham SW, *et al.* Vitamin K and energy transduction: A base strength amplification mechanism. Science 269:1684, 1995.

Dupont HL. Guidelines on acute infectious diarrhea in adults. The Practice Parameters Committee of the American College of Gastroenterology. *Am J Gastroenterol.* 1997, 92: 1962–1975.

F Sizer, E Whitney. "Nutrition Concepts & Controversies"; Brooks Cole; 10th ed., 2005.

Fine KD Diarrhea. In: Feldman M, Scharschmidt BF, Sleisenger MH, *et al.* (eds). Sleisenger & Fordtran's Gastrointestinal and Liver Disease: Pathophysiology/Diagnosis/Management. 6th ed. Philadelphia: Saunders WB, p 128–152, 1998.

Gangarosa RE, Glass RI, Lew JF, *et al.* Hospitalizations involving gastroenteritis in the United States, 1985: The special burden of disease among the elderly. *Am J Epidemiol*, 135: 281–290, 1992.

Garthright WE, Archer DL, Kvenberg JE. Estimates of incidence and costs of intestinal infectious diseases in the United States. Public Health Rep., 103: 107–115, 1988.

Gopalan C, BV Rama Sastri, Balsosubramaniam SC, reprinted. Nutritive Value of Indian Foods. NIN, Hyderabad, 1996.

Gopalan C, Rama Sastri, BV, Balasubramanian SC. Nutritive Value of Indian Foods, National Institute of Nutrition, ICMR, Hyderabad, 1989.

Gopalan C, Ramasastri BV, Balasubramanian SC. Nutritive value of Indian Foods. Revised and updated by Jarasinga Rao BS, Deosthale YG and Pant KC. National Institute of Nutrition, Indian Council of Medical Research, Hyderabad, India, 2000.

Guerrant RL, Van Gilder T, Steiner TS, *et al.* Infectious Diseases Society of America: Practice guidelines for the management of infectious diarrhea. *Clin Infect Dis.*, 32: 331–350, 2001.

Heird WC. Food insecurity, hunger, and undernutrition. In: Kliegman RM, Behrman RE, Jenson HB, *et al.*, (eds). Nelson Textbook of Pediatrics. 18th ed. Philadelphia, Pa: Saunders Elsevier; ch 43, 2007.

Jean-Gerard Pelletier, Children in the Tropics, Severe Malnutrition: A Global Approach, No. 208–209, 1993.

Manay Shakuntala, Shadaksharaswamy M. Foods-Facts and Principles, New Age International (P) Publishers Ltd., Chennai, 1987.

Mosca L, Banka CL, Benjamin EJ, *et al.* Evidence-based guidelines for cardiovascular disease prevention in women: update. *Circulation*, 115:1481–1501, 2007.

Musher DM, Musher BL. Contagious acute gastrointestinal infections. *N Engl J Med.*, 351: 2417–2427, 2004.

Nutrient requirements and recommended dietary allowances for Indians, CM, NIN. Nutrition. Vol. 34. No. 4, Oct. 2000. National Institute of Nutrition. India, 2002.

Nutritional Assessment, RD Lee, DC Neiman. Mosby-Year Book, Inc., St. Louis, 1993.

Park K. Park' s Textbook of Preventive and Social Medicine, Banarsidas Bhanot Publishers, Jabalpur, 482 001, 1995.

Raghuram TC, Parricha Sharma RD. Diet and Diabetes. National Institute of Nutrition. ICMR, 1993.

Rush D. Maternal Nutrition and Perinatal Survival. *Nutr. Rev.* 59:315–326, 2001.

Scheidler MD, Giannella RA. Practical management of acute diarrhea. *Hosp Pract.*, 36: 49–56, 2001.

Schiller LR. Diarrhea. Med Clin North Am., 84: 1259–1274, 2000.

Shearer MJ. Vitamin K. Lancet 345:229, 1995.

Shubhangani Joshi A. Nutrition and Dietetics, Tata McGraw Hill Publishing Co., Ltd., New Delhi, 2002.

Srilakshmi B. Food Science, New Age International, (P) Ltd., Publications, New Delhi, 2003.

Srilakshmi B. Dietetics, New Age International (P) Ltd., New Delhi, 2006.

Srilakshmi B. Food Science, New Age International Private Ltd., New Delhi, 2010.

Sriramachandrasekharan MV, Ravichandran M. Principles of Human Nutrition. Lotus Publishers, Tirunelveli, 1999.

Sriramachandrasekharan MV, Ravichandran M. Principles of Human Nutrition. Lotus Publishers, Tirunelveli, 1999.

Sumati Mudambi R, Shalini Rao M. Food Science, New Age International (P) Publishers Ltd., Chennai, 1989.

Swaminathan M. Essentials of Food and Nutrition, Volume I and II, the Bangalore Printing and Publishing Co. Ltd., Bangalore, 1988.

Thielman NM, Guerrant RL. Acute infectious diarrhea. *N Engl J Med.*, 350: 38–47, 2004.

US Department of Health and Human Services, Healthy People. With Understanding and Improving Health and Objectives for Improving Health. 2 vols 2nd ed, US Government Printing Office Washington DC, 2010.

Vijayapushpam, *et al.* Adolescent Growth Spurt. NIN, Hyderabad, 2008.

Index